THE PRIMORDIAL BREATH

VOLUME I

AN ANCIENT CHINESE WAY OF ATTEMPTING TO PROLONG LIFE THROUGH BREATH CONTROL

Seven treatises from the Taoist Canon, the Tao Tsang, on the esoteric practice of Embryonic Breathing, translated by Jane Huang in collaboration with Michael Wurmbrand.

ORIGINAL BOOKS

Original Books, Inc
PO Box 2948
Torrance, CA 90509, USA

© 1987 by ORIGINAL BOOKS, INC.
All rights reserved.
Second, Revised Edition, 1998.

Printed in the United States of America.
An imprint of Original Books, Inc.
ISBN 0-944558-00-3

TABLE OF CONTENTS

COVER PICTURE TRANSLATIONS, page 5

PREFACE, page 7

SUNG-SHAN T'AI WU HSIEN-SHENG CH'I CHING, page 11
    A Book on Breath by the Master Great Nothing of Sung-Shan.

T'AI HSI CHING CHU, page 41
    The Embryonic Breath Canon, with a Commentary by Huan Chen Hsien Sheng.

T'AI HSI MI YAO KO CHÜEH, page 47
    The Secret Songs about the Embryonic Breath Secret.

T'AI CH'ING FU CH'I K'OU CHÜEH, page 53
    The Extremely Pure Secret Oral Tradition of Breath Ingestion (Attributed to Kuo Chang.)

T'AI CH'ING T'IAO CH'I CHING, page 65
    The Book on the Extremely Pure Harmonizing of The Breath (attributed to Ko Hsien Kung.)

CHEN CH'I HUAN YÜAN MING, page 99
    The Carved (Text) on the Recovery of the Genuine Breath, with a Commentary by Ch'iang Ming Tzu.

CHI KO HSÜAN LAO TZU CHIE CHIE, page 121
    An Edited Text of Ko Hsüan's Commentary to Selections out of Lao Tzu's (Tao Te Ching) by Yen Ling Feng.

GLOSSARY, page 151

BIBLIOGRAPHY, page 171

COVER PICTURE: REPRODUCTION OF A CHOU DYNASTY (500 BC) JADE INSCRIPTION.

(From WILHELM, Hellmut, see Bibliography.)

Hellmut Wilhelm translates it as follows:

"With breathing, proceed as follows: (The breath) should be held and it will be gathered. If it is gathered, it becomes magic. If it becomes magic, it descends. If it descends, it quiets down. If it quiets down, it solidifies. If it is solidified, then it germinates. If it germinates, it grows. If it grows, it is attracted back (upwards.) If it is attracted back, it reaches heavens. In heaven, it still presses up. At the lower end, it still presses down. He who follows this will live; he who acts contrary to this will die."

Kuo Mo-Jo translates it as follows:

"In transporting the breath, the inhalation must be full. When it is full, it has big capacity. When it has big capacity, it can be extended. When it is extended, it can penetrate downward. When it penetrates downward, it will be calmly settled. When it is calmly settled, it will be strong and firm. When it is strong and firm, it will germinate. When it germinates, it will grow. When it grows, it will retreat upward. When it retreats upward, it will reach the top of the head. The secret power of Providence moves above. The secret power of the Earth moves below. He who follows this will live. He who acts against this will die."

The meaning of many of the ideograms of the Chou period is open to interpretation. This is the reason for the different translations. More translated versions of this inscription are published in THE PRIMORDIAL BREATH, Vol. II.

PREFACE

Blue whales are known to live one hundred years and more. For animals of their size, seals and dolphins also enjoy a long life-span. The giant turtle has become legendary as to its longevity. Turtles also hold the record in being able to remain over eight hours under the water, without breathing.

These amazing abilities, shared by all diving animals, could not have remained unnoticed by the Taoists, since they were keen observers of nature. Needham, in his monumental work on science in ancient China, describes the Taoists as the first scientists in human history, who carefully noted down their observations and elaborated theories and methods based upon such observations.

Considering that pearl diving, which started many thousands of years ago in China, was an additional incentive for Chinese to try to imitate nature, it becomes then evident how Taoists related longevity to the capacity to control and stop breathing.

Seventy five percent of the more than 200,000 Chinese pages of the Taoist Canon deal with the subject of long life. The Tao Te Ching of Lao Tzu states that, "the epitome of virtue is to obtain immortality" (Chapter 42, Version A, Ma Wang Tui Excavation.) The Canon, made out of over one thousand six hundred books written in different centuries, deals mainly with this subject. Most of the writings are very abstruse. They use an arcane, multi-level, symbolic language. Many books use alchemical terms, incomprehensible to the researcher who has no access to an esoteric initiation that has been lost since long. However, an extensive body of literature in the Tao Tsang, the Taoist Canon, is explaining in plain language, breathing control practices. The reader will be amazed at the thoroughness and detailed objectivity of the instructions contained in these books.

This volume presents in translation seven of the most intelligible and comprehensive books on the subject. One of the texts dates itself internally toward the end of the eighth century. Two other texts written by Ko Hsüan (also named Ko Hsien Kung) date probably from the beginning of the fourth century. His biography will be found in the glossary. A colophon indicates that one of the books might date from the fourth century A.D. Nothing helpful as to dates was found regarding the other texts or their authors.

A second volume contains translations of less esoteric books in the Canon describing methods to attain long life, including special Taoist gymnastic movements, called Tao-Yin.

Until now, only small portions of the voluminous Taoist Canon have ever been translated. This archaic literature is to this day inaccessible to the average Chinese because of its complexity of subject, language and style. As such, the reader is asked to bear with the translation in passages that seem unclear or even contain contradictions. Due to the abbreviated nature of the Chinese text, additions to it are indicated by parentheses. This is a unique health literature on a practice hardly mentioned outside China. It was researched for the first time by Maspero in the thirties. His book is an excellent primer for this subject as well as for the early medical knowledge of the Chinese.

Though couched in religious terms, the Embryonic Breath practice is more a description of physical exercises than a doctrine. The practitioner tries to store air in his guts, where a transfer of oxygen to the blood seems possible through the intestinal wall. If this takes place, the adept seems to be able naturally to stop breathing for a certain period. The process is claimed to have a good influence upon the general health of the body. It is supposed to cool the body internally and promote good circulation and rejuvenate the skin. The practitioner also gains a peculiar awareness of his body and its workings. This practice was kept secret and the symbolic language used to describe it seems to have found reverberations in the esoteric teachings of other main religions of the world. This will become more evident in the translations presented in the second volume since these texts use a more symbolic language. These other texts also give many more details necessary to the practitioner.

Though the breathing practice described in such greater detail in the different books, is fascinating, the reader, by all means, should reserve his surprise for the last translated text, a unique commentary of Ko Hsüan to passages of Lao Tzu's main work, the Tao Te Ching. One is supposed, of course, to be familiar with this book in *toto*. The interpretation given presents the Tao Te Ching as an arcane text giving breathing control instructions.

A practice outside China, similar to Embryonic Breathing, is the Tibetan Yoga instruction named Dumo or Heat Yoga in which the so-called Vase-Breathing exercise represents the main part of Dumo. In India, it is the practice of Pranayama and particularly that of Kumbakha which appears closest to Embryonic Breathing. While all of the non-Chinese Yoga sources describe such practices vaguely, with hardly any detail beyond a name, Taoist texts on Embryonic Breathing show the writers speaking at great length from personal experience. The books deal extensively with the diet necessary for a successful practice. They explain how breathing is to be trained, refined and even stopped for a time. Also explained are six types of exhalations that may cure diseases and beneficially influence the body internally. **In the Preface to THE PRIMORDIAL BREATH, Volume II, the reader will find an extensive discussion of the different points of this "stop-breathing" method and lengthy quotes on how the six exhalation sounds should be practiced.**

The official record for human retention of breath, consciously undertaken under water, is about thirteen minutes. Seals and whales routinely stop their breathing for over one hour. Modern research on whales and seals has also shown that, while diving, their spleen acts like an oxygen tank. Their spleen releases into the blood stream a significant amount of young red blood cells rich in oxygen. It is, therefore, surprising that all Taoist texts present the spleen as the most important organ in connection with breathing practices. Could indeed such an increased release of young blood cells have a rejuvenating effect on the human body?

The reader should as well be warned not to take lightly, at face value, some of the statements that might seem naive in the light of modern medical knowledge. Due to the distance in time and culture many words, as translated, do not necessarily mean what they appear at first glance to mean. Thus the word "breath" (ch'i) is also conceived as an energy flowing through the body. When one of the texts refers to air escaping out of the lungs otherwise than through the nose or the mouth, it refers probably to a marked increase in perspiration. Most texts under "immortality" understand a long and healthy life. The examples requiring sophistication on the part of the reader are too numerous to be herewith explained. It is hoped, therefore, that the glossary will be helpful.

Lastly, in olden times, the reader of such texts if interested, was supposed to seek and rely on a master's personal pointer in order to achieve effective breath control.

A wish for a long, healthy, meaningful, and happy life is herewith expressed to all those reading this book.

Michael Wurmbrand, October 20th, 1987.

SUNG-SHAN T'AI WU HSIEN-SHENG CH'I CHING
A BOOK ON BREATH BY THE MASTER GREAT NOTHING OF SUNG-SHAN
(Tao Tsang, Vol. xxx, p. 856; Harvard Yenching 569; Wieger 817)

INTRODUCTION

What the bodily form depends on is breath (ch'i) and what breath relies upon is form. When the breath is perfect, the form is perfect (too.) If breath is exhausted, then form dies. Therefore, the scholar who nourishes (his) life refines the form and nourishes (his) breath, so as to nurture his life. No one has form without breath. Consequently, breath and form must be accomplished together. Isn't this evident?

I have been admiring the highest way (TAO) and have been seeking the secret methods in every possible manner. For over thirty years, I have been practicing (the Taoist) breathing and upholding the original true nature. I was not satisfied with what I had heard and seen.

During the years of TA-LI (766-780 A.D.), I met WANG KUNG of the LO-FOU mountain. He came back from the northern mountains. Riding tall and leaning against his whip, he looked at me. I wondered about that unusual person. I induced him to talk. As I expected, he was a superior adept of the way (TAO.) Being moved by my utmost sincerity, he taught me a couple of important breathing methods for body management.

Such kindness is boundless. It is beyond the description of any language. It is said that the important methods of the way (TAO) are not in books. Instead, they are passed down as oral secret methods. The methods of ingesting the breath such as those described in ERH-CHING (the two rays), WU-YA (the five shoots) and LIU-WU (the six wu) deal with the outer breath, which is rigid and hard. It should not be ingested by those who attend to internal nourishing. As for the proper inner breath, it is called the Embryonic Breath. Since it is naturally inside, you do not have to seek outside for it. If you do not have a good teacher's secret oral method, you will work long and hard, yet in vain.

What I have recorded here is the essence (taught by) my teacher along with (my) extended explanations. These are not personal foolish ideas. Once WANG KUNG told me that Lao-Tzu said, "My life depends on me, and not on heaven and earth." (Lao-Tzu) also said, "The heaven, the earth and I share one breath, but each manages it individually. How could heaven and earth put me to death?" These are real and true sayings and important secrets. He who practices breathing must review such three times. I received the teaching respectfully and always practice it with admiration. Those who get by chance (this) secret must be very careful not to teach it or demonstrate it lightly. They should not leak the secret out, otherwise they may encounter disaster.

Chapter I
The Secret of Ingesting Breath

The secret of ingesting breath to cultivate the original true nature is (to be explained) as follows:

Lie down every day, pacify your mind, cut off thoughts and block the breath. Close your fists, inhale through your nose, and exhale through your mouth. Do not let the breathing be audible. Let it be most subtle and fine. When the breath is full, block it. The blocking (of the breath) will make the soles of your feet perspire. Count one hundred times "one and two". After blocking the breath to the extreme, exhale it subtly. Inhale a little more and block (the breath) again. If (you feel) hot, exhale with "Ho". If (you feel) cold, blow the breath out and exhale it with (the sound) "Ch'ui". If you can breathe (like this) and count to one thousand (when blocking), then you will need neither grains nor medicine.

Drink at times a small cup of wine to make the water (saliva) flow pleasantly. If you can count to five thousand (with such blocking), exhalations and inhalations are at your command. The merit (of such breathing) will make itself known: you have the ability to lie down (for long) in water (thus holding your breath, N.T.)

It is important to be persistent when taking in the breath. Only when the genuine breath descends, can you experience the sensation of openness. How can you hope for the magic wings of immortality by indulging in desire and lust? Such matters do not exist.

Even immortals and superior scholars - not to mention ordinary people - cannot attain (immortality) if they do not yet complete their exercise. Simply have faith in the old man's saying: "Practicing it industriously, you will know it surely by yourself."

Chapter II
The Secret of How to Progress in the Mastery (of Breath)

To progress in the mastery (of breath), proceed as follows:

In general, if you desire to ingest breath, you should first secure a high, dry, quiet, and secluded room. It need not be large, but it must be without any wind draft. Inside the room, keep burning incense on the left and right sides; if you do not use Ju-T'ou (term unknown, may be some scenting substance, N.T,) your bed must be thick and soft, and its feet should be slightly elevated. The book Chen Kao states: "A high bed prevents ghosts from blowing." That means that ghosts follow the earth wind to blow on people and perform evil and obstinate acts. The bed should be 3 feet high. There should be an adequate blanket and the pillow should be 3.2 inches high, the lining being 1.9 inches (thick.) The remainder should be level with the back.

Nightly after midnight, when breath is alive, or in the fifth watch (3-5 a.m.) when you are awake from sleep, exhale first with "Ho" the turbid and foul breath from the stomach for nine times. Then stop. However, it is not really necessary to observe the time after midnight or in the fifth watch. Whenever the weather permits it, and you feel harmonious and your stomach is empty, close your eyes, tap your (upper and lower) teeth together 36 times to arouse the soul inside the body. Use both hands to rub your face from your eye sockets up to your left and right ears.

This is the usual procedure a genuine man will be following for TAO-YIN (the Taoist gymnastics.) First ease the joints pleasantly. Then place your tongue as a pillar against the palate, feel the inside of your mouth until the inner and outer saliva juice (flows) in abundance. Swallow it and conduct it to enter the stomach so the soul is pleased with it. (Do it) three times and stop (after each such) three (swallowings.) This means you are rinsing yourself with the magic juice and swallowing (it), to pour upon and irrigate the five viscera. Your face then will brighten up. When you are familiar with the method, the general principle is the same. It is like (following) an adequate and determined plan to liberate the soul, leading the mind to identify with extreme emptiness. The body is like an abandoned reptile skin and the fettered feelings are completely chased away.

Next ingest (the breath.) Close your eyes and clench your fists every time. Only as you release the breath (when exhaling) should you spread out your fingers. Clenching your fists is to close the passages and to guard yourself against evil. A beginner has to practice making the breath and fluid (saliva) flow. Don't clench your fists as yet. After a hundred days, or half a year, when breath is perceived circulating pleasantly and sweat appears on your palms, (only) then clench your fists.

HUANG T'ING CHING (The Yellow Court Canon) says, "Close and block the three frontier passes, (mouth, hands, feet, but also: eyes, nose and mouth, N. T.) delay clenching your fists. Rinse your mouth and swallow the magic juice and the jade flower (saliva.) Then you will not be hungry (ever) and the three worms will die. The mind and the will, will constantly be harmonious. You will attain joy and prosperity."

Chapter III
The Secret of Cultivating the Breath

The secret of cultivating the breath is as follows:

All humans' five viscera have their own respective breath. Lie down at night, close the breath so as to become conscious of being about to ingest breath. Cultivate the breath first in order to make the old food dissolve away so that the breath may exit. (Only) then begin the harmonizing and ingesting (of the breath.)

The method is to close your eyes, clench your fists and lie down with your face upward, your fists placed between the breasts. Draw up both knees and raise your back and buttocks. Firmly block the breath in the sea of breath (the lower TAN T'IEN, N.T) and make it circulate from the inside to the outside, (thus) revolving it. Exhale it with "Ho". Do that 9 times (or)18 times, then stop. This is called "cultivating the Ho breath". After (such exercises), you will be able to harmonize (the breath.)

Chapter IV
The Secret of Harmonizing the Breath

The secret of harmonizing the breath is as follows:

The nose is the heavenly door (while) the mouth is the earthly window. Therefore, inhale through your nose and use your mouth to exhale. Never do otherwise for breath would be in danger and illness would set in. At the same time, exhale and inhale (very) carefully, not allowing any sound to be heard. Do it seven or nine times, so the breath becomes harmonious and peaceful. This is called "harmonizing the breath".

When (this) harmonizing is concluded, then swallow (the breath.) Lie down at night, hold (the breath) so as not to exhale it by the mouth. By constantly willing and persisting, you will attain the harmonizing (of the breath.)

Chapter V
The Secret of Swallowing the Breath

The secret of swallowing the breath is as follows:

The wonder of ingesting the internal breath is in the swallowing of the breath. People confuse the external breath with the internal breath. They can not make the distinction. How very repugnant! Those who do the breathing exercises ought to be careful, because it is atrocious to mistake one breath for the other.

To live, all human beings have received the Original Breath from the heaven and the earth and the Original Breath spreads inside the body and works by itself. Whenever you exhale and swallow, the internal breath and the external breath respond mutually to each other. The internal breath rises straight up from the sea of breath (the lower TAN T'IEN, N.T.) to the throat with the "Ch'ui" (sound.) But when you are about to exhale because of extreme fullness then, on the contrary, you should close your mouth, let it bulge and then swallow it. The sound "Ku, Ku" (will be heard) passing down along your left side. After 20 days (of such practice), a sound like water dripping down a hole may be heard very clearly. In women, it goes down on the right side. The internal breath is thus clearly distinguished from the external breath.

Next, use the will to escort it (down), use your hands to massage it and to send it to the sea of breath, which is three (Chinese) inches under the navel (and) is called the lower TAN T'IEN. In the beginner in breath ingesting, the Shang Chiao (the upper cooking vessel) is still blocked. Use your hands to massage the breath there and to aid it down. When the breath flows, there is no need of massaging anymore.

Three consecutive swallowings (of breath) at one closing of the mouth are called YÜN-HSING (the Cloud Practice.) One wet swallowing is called YÜ-SHIH (the Granting of the Rain.) A beginner's breath is not thoroughly flowing yet; you must just practice the Yü-Shih or Yün-Hsing for each swallowing. Do not rush to achieve three consecutive (swallowings.) When the breath flows pleasantly, then increase slightly (the number of swallowings) to obtain "a small achievement". After one year, you will be able to swallow breath at will without impediment. If your breath does not flow (properly) or does not go down, you must limit yourself to one swallowing. For every swallowing, when the breath is extremely full, let your mouth bulge greatly and use a little strength to contract it and swallow the breath. Be sure to have the subtle sound of the flowing (in the lower abdomen which sounds like) "Ku Ku". The breath enters then straight into the sea of breath.

After this, you may do three consecutive swallowings. This is how (the proficiency) is properly achieved. Moreover, the secret here is to benefit one's own body. One should swallow the breath deeply. Those who do not practice with concentrated effort for a long time will not be able to compare, evaluate and see the truth of this genuine principle.

It is very fortunate to obtain the breathing secret here for the beginner in swallowing breath as well as for the one (who has been) practicing for long, and not obtaining its wonder yet. How fortunate (they are.)

To teach (this secret) indiscreetly to others will be cause for reprimand and punishment. Be careful! Be careful! During each practice (session), face EAST. When you reach the end, start all over always from the beginning. The proper way is to practice according to the aforementioned method.

Chapter VI
The Secret of Guiding the Breath

The secret of guiding the breath is as follows:

There are two points on the spine behind the lower TAN T'IEN. They correspond through the ridge vein with the NI WAN (MUD PILL) which is the brain palace (a point between the eyes above the root of the nose, N.T.)

The Original Breath is obtained by storing (the breath of) every three consecutive swallowings in the lower TAN T'IEN. Use the mind to take (the Original Breath) in and to make it enter the two points. (You should) imagine two columns of white breath going straight up on both sides of your spine and entering the NI WAN to becloud thickly the palace. Then the breath continues to your hair, your face, your neck, both arms and hands up and to your fingers. After a little time, it enters the chest and the middle TAN T'IEN which is (by) the heart. It pours on into the five viscera, it passes the lower TAN T'IEN, and reaches SAN-LI (the Three Miles, i.e. the genitals, N.T.) It goes through your hips, your knees, ankles and all the way to the YÜNG CH'ÜAN (acupuncture points) which are in the center of your feet soles. That is the so-called "to share one breath and manage it individually".

Then, "the thunder drums, or the moistening by wind and rain" means that, though there are springs in the world, the air cannot moisten and refresh the ten thousand things unless thunder acts. Similarly, although there are saliva and fluids in the human body, they cannot irrigate the five viscera unless one rinses (the mouth) and swallows the saliva. The brilliancy of the restoring of the essence to nourish the brain will not happen, unless there is an encounter (of the saliva and the body fluids.) For swallowing and ingesting, the internal breath cannot be pumped up and used, unless there is breathing. Understanding beforehand the revolving and unfolding of the way (TAO) and the principle of using it, is the way to imitate heaven and earth. Think that the turbid, evil, coagulated and obstructed bad air as well as the stale and coagulated blood are cleansed and removed by this authentic breath and they are expelled from your hands, feet and fingertips. This is called the dispersing of the breath. Extend your fingers. You do not have to clench your fists. One such (practice) period corresponds to one circulation (of the breath.)

When circulating like this, the breath may be lumpy. If it becomes lumpy, you must harmonize it again to make it even. If it is even, then bulge (your mouth) and swallow (the breath) as before. Shut up the breath, bulge (your mouth), then swallow the breath and continue till (you) reach thirty-six swallowings. This is what is referred to as a "small accomplishment". At this time, you have not cut out (eating) grains yet, but you must eat only a little to make your stomach spacious, empty, and clean. Whether sitting or lying down, whenever your stomach is empty, swallow (the air.) Throughout the night you can reach ten times (36 swallowings.) This would make three hundred and sixty swallowings and is called "the great accomplishment". (The result) is called the Great Embryonic Breath. When (you achieve) the Embryonic Breath, shut it off and count up to one thousand two hundred breaths (while blocking the breath.) This is also called a "great accomplishment". If you are unable to refine the form and transform the material substance, though you may accomplish (in some way) the prolongation of life, you will remain identical to a withered log lacking (its natural) splendor.

You will find below the following topics: The refining, the closing, the discarding and the spreading of the breath, and (other) miscellaneous matters. I am going to list the essential secrets below. Those superior men of the same aspiration should practice them carefully. They shall not miss one merit in ten thousand.

Chapter VII
The Secret of How to Refine the Breath

The secret of refining the breath is as follows:

To ingest the breath, go into a room, undress, loosen your hair, lie down face up, stretch out your hands, don't tighten the fists, comb your hair thoroughly and let it fall down and spread it out on the mat. Harmonize then the breath and swallow it. After that, close the breath in and hold it to the extreme. Then darken the mind and shut off any thought. Let the breath go to every vein. When you feel absolutely stuffy, exhale (the breath.) If you are panting, harmonize it. Wait for the breath to become even. Refine it again in the same manner. When it flows freely, increase then such holdings of the breath to reach twenty, thirty, forty, fifty consecutive times. Then the entire body will perspire. This phenomenon is the verification (of success.) At this point, your mind is quiet and the breath is harmonious. You should just lie down, do not get up and rush into the draft. This is a good method to get rid of aging and to prolong life. Practice this when your mind is clear and your breath comfortable. Do not do it when (you are) sleepy. Keep doing the (above practice) but not necessarily each day. Do it only when you are feeling good and comfortable. The proper measure is to do it once every five or ten days. HUANG T'ING CHING (the Yellow Court Canon) states, "A thousand calamities are removed and a hundred diseases are cured. Not only one is not afraid of the tiger's and the wolf's ferocity, one's aging is also banished and life is, therefore, prolonged." This is the secret.

Chapter VIII
The Secret of Discarding the Breath

The secret of discarding the breath is as follows:

In order to discard the breath, the breath and the body have to be harmonious and peaceful, the mind and the soul have to be at ease and smooth. It can be done regardless of sitting down or lying down. Harmonize the breath according to the "door" and the "window" (nose and mouth method.) Whether you are in bed or sitting on a chair, you look thoughtless, still and tranquil. Make the mind identical to the great void. Undertake then to shut off ten or twenty breathings. Make sure there is no wrangling between the breath and the will. After a long time, the breath will exit naturally through the hundreds of hair pores rather than be exhaled. There may still be 10-20% (of the normal) breathing. Harmonize (the breath) again till you can reach 100% of such held-up breathings. If you can hold more than one hundred breathings, you can increase (the number.) Persist in the practice whether walking, standing, sitting or lying down. Just keep doing it diligently. The hundred joints then open up and communicate, the complexion is enriched and made pleasant, the breath is purified and prolonged as after a good bath.

Then you do it whenever the body is not harmonious. You will feel refreshed and pleasant. HUANG T'ING CHING (the Yellow Court Canon) states, "Respecting non-action, both the (upper) HUN and the (lower) P'O souls are peaceful. (My) clean and pure soul appears and converses with me." That is it.

Chapter IX
The Secret of Closing the Breath

The secret to close is as follows:

If suddenly there is discomfort in cultivating and nourishing (the breath) or occasionally there is some kind of illness, go into a secluded room and follow this method: spread out your hands and feet, then harmonize the breath and swallow it down (guiding it in your thoughts) to where the trouble is. Shut off the breath. Use the will and the mind to regulate the breath in order to attack the ailment. When the breath has been retained to the extreme, exhale it. Then swallow it again. If the breathing is rapid, stop. If the breath is harmonious, work on the ailment again. Twenty, thirty, forty, or fifty times, attack where you feel the ailment. If perspiration appears and you feel (you are) communicating and nourished, then stop. If the ailment is not cured, then will to work on it often on a daily basis at midnight or perhaps in the fifth watch (3-5 a.m.) or during the daytime, until there is a difference. Even if the ailment is in your head, face, hands or feet, wherever it is, work on it. There is nothing that will not be cured. Note that when the mind wills the breath into the limbs, it works like magic, its effects are indescribable.

Chapter X
The Secret of Spreading the Breath

The secret of spreading the breath is as follows:

If you use the breath to cure people's diseases, first examine the patient (to find out) which one of the five viscera is sick. The healer has to attempt to disperse the proper, corresponding breath inside the patient's body. Make the patient face the proper direction and quiet him down until (he is) thoughtless. Spreading the breath this way cures the patient. Then (have him) swallow the breath and stop thoughts in order to remove (the sickness.) The evil breath is naturally cut off forever (while) the genuine breath spreads out until the evil air withdraws naturally.

Chapter XI
The Secret of the Six (Types of) Exhalations

(Detailed explanations given by MASPERO regarding the six methods of exhalations are reproduced in the Preface to THE PRIMORDIAL BREATH volume II. N.T.)

The secret of the six (types of) exhalations is as follows (the subscript indicates the pronouncing tone of each Chinese ideogram, N.T.)

The six breathings are: HSI_4, HO_1, HU_1, $HSÜ_1$, $CH'UI_1$, and HSI_1. Each of the five viscera depends on one of these breathings. The additional (the sixth) is for the three cooking vessels. Thus, all are accounted for.

The HSI_4 breathing belongs to the lungs which rule the nose. If you feel blocking heat, lack of harmony and immense exhaustion, then rely on the HSI_4 breathing. Likewise, if your skin is ulcerated, painful or sick, rely on this to work on it and it will heal immediately.

The **HO₁** breathing belongs to the heart which is ruling the tongue. If (your tongue) is dry and rough and if your breath is bad and does not flow freely, then do the **HO₁** breathing to expel it. If there is a great amount of heat, open up your mouth completely, (but) for a small amount of heat, open it up slightly. You must pay attention to properly judge the situation and manage the **HO₁** breathing. Disobeying this principle would for sure injure you.

The **HU₁** breathing belongs to the spleen which rules CHUNG KUNG T'U (the central palace territory, the abdomen.) If your breath is slightly hot and inharmonious, if your stomach feels sick, filled, stuffy and constipated, then it is to be handled with the **HU₁** breathing to heal (it.)

The **HSÜ₁** breathing belongs to the liver which rules the eyes. If your eyes are warm or hot, you may use the **HSÜ₁** breathing to handle them and heal them.

The **CH'UI₁** breathing connects with the kidneys which rule the ears. If your loins and feet are cold and your genitals are declining, use the **CH'UI₁** breathing to handle and heal them.

The **HSI₁** breathing belongs to the three cooking vessels. If (they are) inharmonious, then use the **HSI₁** breathing to handle them.

Though the six breathings have their respective territories, when the five viscera and the three cooking vessels are hot or cold to the utmost, or they lack harmony, use the **HO₁** breathing to heal (them) since they are all connected to the heart. It is not necessary to use the (other) breathings.

All sects agree that when this method (the **HO₁** breathing) is practiced, the efficacy of the cure can be observed immediately.

Chapter XII
The Secret of Harmonizing the Saliva

The secret of harmonizing the saliva is as follows:

Man eats the five flavors. Each one of the five flavors corresponds to one of the five viscera. The foul breath of each of the viscera is exhaled through the mouth. Moreover, the breaths of the six receptacles (stomach, gall bladder, large and small intestines, the bladder and the three cooking vessels counted as one, N.T.) and of the three cooking vessels (separately) also gather at this common opening (the mouth.)

All uncleanness collects and becomes foul breath. Every time you wake up, the turbid breath is naturally unbearable to the smell. If you are careful, you should know its time. When your mouth is dry, your tongue rough, your cheeks hot, and there is (too) little saliva, or you cannot eat because of a sore throat: it is heat. You should open your mouth and exhale with the HO_1 breathing. Do it by the proper "door" and "window" (nose and mouth method.) For each ten HO_1 (exhalations or) twenty HO_1 (exhalations) sound the heavenly drum (tap the upper and lower teeth together, N.T.) perhaps seven or nine (times.) Use your tongue to rinse the flowery pond (saliva) and swallow the saliva. Repeat the HO_1, breathing. Observe whether the heat has subsided. The heart is in good condition only when the fresh fluid and the sweet spring are produced in the mouth. When the heat is gone, the five viscera are cool. If the saliva is cold and (yet) not juicy, it is due to coldness. Use then the $CH'UI_1$ breathing to cure (this condition.) Then when the inside of your mouth is tasting good naturally and the mind is harmonious, stop.

HUANG T'ING CHING (the Yellow Court Canon) states, "The clear water of the jade pond pours down to the magic root. Be careful to nourish it and you may live long."

It says also, "Calamities will not invade him who rinses (his mouth) and swallows the magic fluid"

Chapter XIII
The Secret of Drinking and Eating

The secret of drinking and eating is as follows:

After ingesting breath, when the nourishing is orderly, you may eat. Some food can be harmful, some can be beneficial. You should eat what is beneficial and cut out on what is harmful. You should always take what is good.

Every morning, eat some well-boiled flavorless rice porridge; this will manage properly the spleen breath and activate satisfactorily the saliva. At noon, eat plain flour dough boiled in water. It is good. So are thick onions or shallots soup, cooked glutinous rice or barley, and dried shredded deer meat (a Chinese way of meat conservation, N.T.). After eating, swallow three to five grains of raw pepper. First swallow the breath for 3 to 5 swallowings to disperse the food and to make it pass down. The pepper makes the breath flow harmoniously to the three cooking vessels and the five viscera. It overcomes the foul breath and helps the genuine breath. The pepper is especially good when taken on a long term basis. It can ward off coldness, heat, or humidity, clear up eyesight, harmonize body systems, and manage breath. Its merits are too numerous to be all listed.

The first volume of T'AI CH'ING CHING (The Great Purity Book) elucidates more wonderful methods. Avoid eating the meat of the 12 astrological animals or the thirty-six creatures (see Glossary) as they are the root of life as is a father or a mother. Avoid hot steamed buns as they disturb the correct breathing. Fat pork and raw vegetables block the human arteries. Gourds, jujube, chestnut, taro, water caltrop, the foxnut (Euryale Ferox), the meat of the hornless river deer, the wild goose as well as wild fowl may be eaten except for their heart, head, and fat. If you fast, you must interrupt (the above diet.)

What T'IEN SHI (CHANG TAO LING) planted was the Jade (jewel) of all plants. It is named the NAN CHU TS'AO (LI-MU - the Southern Candle Grass or ANDROMEDA OVALIFOLIA - N.T.) Each bush grows seventy-two stalks. Each stalk grows twenty-four branches. Each branch has five leaves. The numbers correspond exactly to the seventy-two HOU (periods, the five-day periods in the 360-day year), the five elements, and the twenty-four CH'I (periods of 15 days each.) (This plant) is to be found east of the YANGTZE RIVER by the SHAO SHIH Mountain, along the NAN YUE. It can also be found by the HSIANG RIVER and HUA CHUNG. It is good to be eaten cooked together with rice. It is also good fried in oil. It is not necessary to follow exactly what is required by the Great Purity Book. One can take the NAN CHU TS'AO alone.

Whenever you eat, it is better not to eat to the full since fullness will injure your heart and the breathing practice will be difficult. Avoid thick soups of turnips, or radishes and vegetables that are raw, cold, and pungent. What is sour, slimy, sticky, greasy, stale, hard, or difficult to digest is quite forbidden. If, by accident, you take a bite of such food, there will be some subtle pain wherever (such food) stays (inside the body.) Be careful! Be careful! Eat without any apprehension only soft food. In general, after ingesting the breath, if there is gas, let it go down and leak out. Do not try to stop that. If you stop such, you will get sick.

Each morning, with an empty stomach, just follow your natural disposition and drink one tiny cup of good, clear wine, which is to be warmed up in winter and may be cool during the summer. It helps the main correct breath expel the evil breath. Do not over-drink since you would get inebriated and this would injure your soul and the possibility of a long life. If you meet with honored guests and you cannot help but have to drink, then breathe out with the HO_1 (exhalation) 3 to 5 times. If you have to drink more than one cup at a time, open your mouth and breathe out with **HO₁** over ten times to expel the poison of fermentation. When commonly trained in this practice, the person who usually drinks only two, three liters (of wine) daily can drink ten without becoming inebriated. Even without having eaten first, he will not be overcome and will behave as usual.

Chapter XIV
The Secret of Nurturing

The secret of nurturing is as follows:

Whenever you are nourishing, refining and ingesting the breath, the way (to avoid foul air) is to avoid attending a birth or ascending into a funeral parlor. Moreover, do not even smell the bad air of the six types of dead cattle, all that is rotten, unclean, impure, any horse or dirty things, let alone approach such. If you see something ominous, stinking or unclean, you must chant an incantation to get rid of such uncleanness; otherwise, it is extremely injurious to the genuine breath. Should you happen upon such uncleanness unexpectedly, then shut off the breath immediately, and seek the upwind to move on and get away from it fast. It is good to clean and wash out well (the foul smell by drinking) two cups of wine. If the foul breath penetrates (inside you) and (you) perceive (yourself) unsettled and insecure, you must harmonize the breath to get rid (of the foul air) so it will not remain. In addition, there might be adverse breath (eructations, N.T.) Then you should not let the breath come out, but, on the contrary, swallow it and inhale the breath to counteract it. Be sure to help ease it out by rubbing your upper abdomen with your hand. Keep some pepper grains in your mouth and drink one or two cups of wine to disperse (the adverse breath.) (As long as) it is not dispersed, you cannot (feel) harmonious and peaceful. The above (rebellious breath) must have come from having eaten greasy food which disturbs and harms the main correct breath. Examine yourself carefully. Then you should know what your previous offenses were. If they are sadness, anger, or sex, do not allow those to impede (the practice) again.

After you have been ingesting the breath for a whole year, it will flow; after the second year, it will circulate; after the third year, the virtue is achieved: the Original Breath is completed and it coagulates into a dark (mysterious) pearl in the elixir field (TAN T'IEN.) At that point, even in case there would be offenses, they could not cause calamity.

Swallow one thousand swallowings every day and do not be afraid it might be too much. As a result, (this practice) will reverse what is old and restore youth. The reversal (phenomenon) starts (with this practice.) Then, the breath transforms into blood, the blood transforms into essence (or sperm), the essence transforms into marrow. The breath is transformed in the first year. The blood is transformed in the second year. The blood arteries are transformed in the third year. The flesh is transformed in the fourth year. The marrow is transformed in the fifth year. The sinews are transformed in the sixth year. The bones are transformed in the seventh year. The hair is transformed in the eighth year. The body is transformed in the ninth year. Within ten years, the thirty-six thousand spirits perfect the body so that it be transformed into an immortal who genuinely (deserves) to be called a SHEN-JEN (genie.)

The man who zealously nourishes the utmost way (TAO) refines breath into form. The form is transformed into the soul, and the soul and form are united. Then he can ascend to heavens in broad daylight. That is the great way's (TAO) magic manifestation.

Those who want to be immortals should learn carefully and persistently. As a consequence, (their) nature opens up to communicate and their five viscera strengthen each other mutually.

HUANG T'ING CHING (The Yellow Court Canon) states, "Thousands and hundreds will naturally be connected. Ones and tens will be arranged like rows of mountain ranges". That is it.

(When one's) inside breath does not exit and the outside air does not enter, cold or heat will not affect (one) and a soldier's sword will not injure (one.) Being transformed and ascending (to heavens), one has long life identical to the three brilliant (ones) (the sun, the moon, and the stars - N.T.) It is entirely inexhaustible.

Chapter XV
The Secret of Ceasing (to Eat) Grains

The secret of discontinuing (the feeding on) grains is as follows:

(When you want) to cease feeding on grains, (you should) rely only upon the efforts to nourish (the breath) as formerly (described.) At the end of three years of industrious nourishing, the genuine breath flows freely, the body is solid and the bones are full (with marrow.) Hundreds of souls are keeping their positions, and the Three Corpses (in the three elixir fields, N.T.) flee away. In this way, gradually there is no desire to smell the aroma of the five flavors. There is constant thinking of not wanting to eat. When your eating must be ceased, let it be ceased. It is not difficult anymore. Whenever you feel your belly empty, you must swallow breath, whether it is morning or evening, regardless of any limit. After a long time, you will naturally become harmonious. It is not necessary to annoy you with all the details of conditions and timing.

Moreover, you may, at the same time, take medicine. Most people only take medicine and do not swallow breath. During their short life span, they are concerned only with the medicine. Therefore, they do not reach the goal. It is not a superior scholar's way to use (his) mind.

HUANG T'ING CHING (The Yellow Court Canon) states: "The grains of hundreds of cereals are the spirits of the earth. Though the five flavors are beautiful on the outside, they (actually) are an evil foul-smelling demon. The foul smell corrupts the soul and the Embryonic Breath is annihilated. How can you attain the return of infancy? Why not eat breath which is the supreme harmonious essence, so as to be able not to die and enter the HUANG NING (The Yellow Repose)?"

Chapter XVI
The Secret of Being Careful and Genuine

The secret of being careful and genuine is as follows:

People in this world generally have various intense desires and passions (which) injure life and cut short (their) destinies. It has been like this since ancient times. Regrets are to no avail if it is not prevented.

HSIEN CHING (A book on immortality) says: "(Only) when facing death do men begin to treasure (their) bodies. Only after crime has been committed do they think of moving towards goodness. (When) faced with suffering, (then they) strive to seek medicine." The natural abilities have been dissipated. How can they be sought after and retrieved?

Therefore, the able, the wise and the scholars treasure life when it is not yet endangered. They are careful about a calamity before it happens. They cure the ailment before it comes. Hence, they shake off the worldly clothes (of vice) and pacify the mind to return to the way (TAO.) The way (TAO) is breath. The ruler of the body is the essence (sperm, N.T.) This essence is the root of life. By cherishing the essence and treasuring the breath, you are likely to prolong life."

HUANG T'ING CHING (The Yellow Court Canon) states: "Think of the arcane viscera within the square inch (the NI WAN point, N.T.) Restore the three spirits (of the three TAN T'IEN) to revert old age into strength." It also says, "Be careful to the utmost of hurried sex (if you wish) to prolong life. Why be dead and make your soul weep silent tears? When the three divine souls are neglected and die, you go to the land of calamity. You should inhale breath and retain the essence (or sperm.) The one inch (square) field (THE NI WAN, N.T.) in the one-foot dwelling (the face, N.T.) is able to manage life. Hundreds of rivers collapse if dikes of the sea break. When leaves fall off, the tree withers and loses its lustrous green."

This is the way to retain and nourish the essence. In learning to prolong life, it is impossible to learn to prolong life without cherishing the essence (sperm) and nourishing the breath. Everybody knows of the way (TAO) of YIN TAN PAI YU (the hundred ways to protect the YIN elixir (a Taoist sexual practice, N.T.). However, even though a man devotes attention to breath, without abandoning lust, he still cannot avoid (at the same time) danger (to himself.) It is said therefore, "It is man who constantly loses the way (TAO), it is not the way (TAO) that loses man. It is man who always abandons the way (TAO), the way (TAO) does not abandon man." The superior person who is nourishing (the breath) should think and examine himself carefully.

Breath is TAO (principle, or way.) TAO is emptiness and non-being. Emptiness and non-being is nature (itself.) Nature is non-action (WU WEI.) Non-action is the non-moving of the mind. The non-moving of the mind means that there is no starting inside the mind. If there is no starting inside the mind, then the outside state (of mind) does not enter. When internal and external tranquillity is attained, the soul is accomplished. If the soul is accomplished, then breath is harmonious. If breath is harmonious, then the Original Breath comes naturally. If the Original Breath comes naturally, then the five viscera are nourished and moist. When the five viscera are nourished and moist, hundreds of channels flow and communicate. If hundreds of channels flow and communicate, then the saliva comes up in response. When the saliva comes, then there is no need for the five flavors. If the five flavors are stopped and dispensed with, hunger or thirst will not occur. When hunger and thirst do not occur, the Three Fields accomplish the body. The bones are strong; the flesh, solid. Hence, old age is reversed, years regress. The transformation starts then. Consequently, breath transforms into blood. The blood transforms into essence (or sperm.) The essence transforms into marrow. In the first year, the breath is changed. In the second year, the blood is changed. In the third year, the channels are changed. In the fourth year, the flesh is changed. In the fifth year, the marrow is changed. In the sixth year, the tendons are changed. In the seventh year, the bones are changed. In the eighth year, the hair is changed. In the ninth year, the body is changed.

These thirty-six thousand souls (spirits) reside inside the body. One is transformed into an immortal. The mind is able to understand the mysterious subtle and to manage the unexpected. The five viscera will be in harmony. The saliva is produced. The three (cooking) vessels open up, breath is unobstructed. This is called CH'IUNG TAN (the best of elixirs.) It is not the worldly elixir. The soul is the utmost magic of non-form. The soul is naturally endowed with the Way (TAO.) It is quiet and identical to nature.

Man is naturally endowed with a soul. When he moves, he conforms with the circumstances. Therefore, when man follows nature, his soul coagulates (taking form.) If it lasts for a long time, the soul stays without moving. If disturbed, the soul flees. If the soul stays without moving, man is alive, but should the soul flee, man dies. This is caused by changing circumstances, not by the soul.

(When you) want to ingest breath, you must first quietly sit through one session. After you consciously transcend the world of sensuous desires, the form and the formless realm of pure spirit, you go past the ultimate origin, the extreme plainness, the extreme beginning, the grand ultimate (T'AI CHI) and the extreme heights. Think that the Original Breath comes down from the top door and enters. Will it to enter the Yüng Ch'üan points (the bubbling springs, acupuncture points on the soles.) Sit up (in meditation), count the number of the entering breaths but not of the exhalations. Use only one awakening to lead and will the Original Breath to (make it) arrive to the three TAN T'IEN. It revolves like a flowing stream.

WANG LAO CHING (The Old Ruler Book) states "If the Original Breath flows and communicates, a superior (adept) knows the TAO (principle) of non-death. It is not worthwhile to discuss it with inferior people." Be careful! It also states, "By doing the Embryonic Breathing and guarding the center, you will be able to be connected to the heaven above. It is called the great way (TAO.) Practice this and the flight to immortality will be obtained immediately." Keep (this principle) secret, be careful with it, protect it!

Chapter XVII
The Secret of the Nourishing and Preserving

The way to do the Embryonic Breathing is as follows:

Start the practice with taping your teeth (together) thirty-six times (so as) to summon all the spirits together. Next, turn your neck around (like a turtle) for one round. (Make circular movements with your head, inclining it on all sides, N.T.) The Embryonic Breath involves swallowing down the breath. Swallow three times in this way. Then guide your tongue to go past the entire front and back sides of your teeth to obtain the jade saliva until it fills your mouth; rinse (your mouth) with it and then tilt your head backwards and swallow the saliva.

Above, it repairs the NI WAN (the mud-pill point between the eyebrows, N.T.); below, it moistens the five viscera.

At midnight and in the fifth night watch (3-5 a.m.), stretch out your feet, tighten your fists, (place) both hands (about) five inches away from the body; the pillow (should be) about three inches (high); shut your eyes and follow the previously described method of swallowing.

After combing and washing yourself, warm up one cup of wine and drink it. The Embryonic Breath nourishes the six receptacles. The wine leads the breath into moistening the hundred joints.

A wise man said, "Man (is) inside the breath, breath is inside man. If man does not separate from breath, breath does not separate from man. Man depends on breath to be alive, for when breath is dissipated, man dies." The principle of man's life and death is entirely based on breath. By harmonizing and refining the Original Breath, should (man) even seek death he would not be able to find it."

WANG LAO said, "Practicing (breath ingesting) for a long time, death, even if sought after, could not be obtained." This is what it means.

LAO CHÜN said, "The sweet rain moistens the ten thousand things, the Embryonic Breath moistens the hundred bones."

HUANG T'ING CHING (The Yellow Court Canon) states, "(Nourish) day and night without sleeping, (and) one will become an immortal."

At its best, it brings immortality, and at the very least, it profits toward long life. If the body is sick, meditate on breath (so as) to work on the illness and the sickness will be healed promptly.

When the genuine breath drives away the turbid breath to leak out below, then one will be in a happy, high spirit and filled with harmonious charisma.

LAO CHÜN said, "The magic valley and the jade flower are (to be found) in your own body." To try and pluck medicinal plants in famous mountains or great marshes and to take such medicine may nourish and assist the right breath. But if you depend entirely on the medicine, it is against the way (TAO.) If you ingest constantly the Embryonic Breath for a long time, the breath will mature naturally and achieve genuine wonder. Without depending on feathery wings, you will fly up quickly.

An embryo is a baby who tightens its fists and swallows the Original Breath. The fist-tightening is (the closing) of the space between heaven and earth. It is like the mind closing its door to prevent the foul breath. The baby tightens its fists inside (its) mother's womb in order to swallow its Original Breath. Therefore, this is called the Embryonic Breath. It contains the Original Breath as a root. Immovable and unshakable, the baby is thus naturally free from hunger and thirst. (As) you learn the Original Embryonic Breath by blocking breathing when you feel the stuffiness caused by the blocking, you may exhale the dirty air subtly by using the "Ho_1" exhalation to expel it.

You will then soon resume blocking. Being constantly on your guard for the Original, you will naturally achieve (its) wonder.

The human body is given life by receiving the Original Breath. It still needs the Original Embryonic Breath to nurture it. (This practice) is therefore called "Preserving (one's) Original Breath." It is (also) called "The Natural Restoring of the Elixir." PU HSÜ said, "The harmonious breath soars into the void. Exhale and inhale the breath of the glowing clouds. The Embryonic Breath will calm down hundreds of joints. Quietly investigate the three conveniences (spirit, breath, essence or sperm, N.T.) The NI WAN (Palace) will illuminate the bright mirrors. The golden flower of immortality is thus achieved."

It was also said, "Think constantly of ingesting the original essence. Through the refining of the fluid, you solidify the form and the substance."

The man of the way (TAO) constantly retains the Original Breath. He draws out the saliva and rinses in his mouth the glowing mist to fill up and irrigate joints and palaces. The saliva moistens your bones and joints and reverses the withering and rotting old age, so that you have the pleasant complexion of the young. To transform the complexion through breathing, if the saliva is not refined like this before the Original Breath rushes against the throat, how can you respond? Respond with the thunder sound. That is the Embryonic Breath. Fist tightening will also do. Beneath the throat is the twelve storied tower, (the trachea, N.T.) In the Embryonic Breath (system), breath communicates up to the head. The swallowing is called the method to nurture the brain. Keep it secret. For it was said, "When hungry, eat the extremely harmonious natural breath. This is the Embryonic Breath. When thirsty, drink the nectar of the flowery pond. That is the saliva inside the mouth."

Bring up the saliva and return it to irrigate the gates of the soul. Thus, the palaces of the kidneys are nourished and enriched, and the jade juice is sweet. This (secret) is to be kept.

The five viscera correspond to the arrangement of the stars above; below, (they) correspond to the five elements. Keep (them) constantly clear and pure.

Chapter XVIII
The Method of Breathing Carefully

The method of breathing carefully is as follows:

It is within the nature of breathing to have difficulty in retaining the inhalation while the exhalation is easily exhausted. What is difficult to retain is to be guarded whole. What is easily exhausted should be well kept and prevented from leaking out.

An immortal said, "To learn the way (TAO) is like recalling what you have eaten in the morning. It is not impossible to do. To treasure breath is like loving your face and your eyes. It has never been unattainable."

It was also said, "I rarely see (someone) withering and haggard when he makes his treasuring of breath a top priority." Be thrifty of talking and laughing. When doing exercises, it is especially proper not to shout out too loud. Similarly do other things carefully to avoid injury.

Man, heaven and earth are identical. The changes of the mixed breath of Yin and Yang, the skin, the bones, the marrow, the receptacles, the viscera, blood, breath, the exhalation and the inhalation, advancement or withdrawal, cold or heat or other variables, all are identical to the two instruments (heaven and earth) and the five elements. One knows therefore that when the breath of Yin and Yang is in disarray, heaven and earth do not prosper. When the viscera and the receptacles are not harmonized, the veins and channels will be ill. This is because the pains of the outside cold and heat are stirred up by the wind. Hundreds of illnesses are provoked by breath. That is why it was said, "The genuine breath comes after a quiet and insipid voidness. If the essence and the soul are protecting the inside, how could illnesses come?" You must therefore know the form and the soul according to nature. Harmonize and perfect them. Investigate the causes of internal and external illnesses and pay attention to them.

Man has three elixir fields (TAN T'IEN) which contain the Three Originals: the upper (one), the middle (one) and the lower (one.) The upper one is the NI WAN (Mud Pill), or brain palace. Its spirit is a red child, alias YÜEN HSIEN (The Original First), or TI-CH'ING (The Imperial Lord.) The spirit wears red clothes and a red cap and it governs the Upper Capital. The middle Elixir Field (TAN T'IEN) is the crimson palace, the heart. Its immortal is named TZU-TAN (The Elixir Boy), alias CHUNG KUANG CHIEN (The Firm, Brilliant Center.) The spirit wears a red mantle and cap and it rules the Middle Capital. The lower Elixir Field (TAN-T'IEN) is situated below the navel in the sea of breath. It is the gate of the essence (or sperm.) Its spirit is The Baby, alias YÜAN-YANG (The Original Yang), or KU-HSIA (The Lower Valley.) (It wears) a dark red mantle and cap and it rules the Lower Capital.

These are the three Elixir Fields (TAN T'IEN), each corresponding to one of the three capitals, with one spirit each. If they are weak or impaired, then the breath leaks out and the essence pours down. If the essence pours down, then the breath scatters. This essence is the root of the body. This root is the seat of the breath. If the essence is intact, then the breath is perfected. If the essence leaks out, then the breath (also) leaks out. It is necessary that the essence and the breath should be intact. It was also said, "The essence is able to feed on the breath. The form is able to feed on the (five) flavors."

When swallowing breath, do not do it along with the saliva. The saliva should be swallowed separately. If (it is swallowed) along with the saliva, there is the danger of raw air entering the stomach and causing illness. In swallowing the saliva, wait till the breath is exhaled. This (turns out to be) especially wonderful.

The end of the SUNG-SHAN T'AI WU HSIEN-SHENG CH'I CHING.

T'AI HSI CHING CHU
THE EMBRYONIC BREATH CANON, WITH A COMMENTARY
BY HUAN CHEN HSIEN SHENG
(Tao Tsang Vol. IV, p. 206; Harvard Yenching 59; Wieger 127)

THE EMBRYO IS COAGULATED OUT OF THE INSIDE BREATH.

The sea of breath lies three inches below the navel. It is also (called) the lower Tan T'ien (the elixir field.) It is also (called) the dark female (Hsüan-P'in.) People usually say that Hsüan-P'in is the mouth and the nose. That is wrong. The mouth and the nose are the entering and exiting doors for Hsüan-P'in. The word "Hsüan" means (also) water, and the word "P'in" means mother. It is known in the world that the Yin and Yang breaths meet and coagulate, (originating) from a (father's) water (sperm) and a mother. It becomes an embryo within three months. The form is completed in ten months and has become a human being. Those who are practicing the nourishing way (TAO), store the breath beneath the navel and keep their soul inside their body. Soul and breath combine together and produce the mysterious embryo. Once the mysterious embryo is conceived, it will produce a body by itself. This is the inner elixir and the way (TAO) of non-death.

THE BREATH GROWS INSIDE THE EMBRYO.

The soul is the child of the breath, and breath is the mother of the soul. Soul and breath follow each other just as form and shadow do. The moment there is coagulation in the mother's womb, the child-spirit grows naturally. This is to say that the Original Breath will not be dissipated.

WHEN BREATH COMES IN THE BODY, IT IS CALLED LIFE. IF THE SPIRIT DEPARTS THE FORM, IT IS (CALLED) DEATH.

The Hsi Sheng Canon states, "A person's body is growing for (his) soul to reside (in it) and the soul is the lord of the body. If the host human being is anxious and moving, the soul will leave. If the soul leaves, then breath disperses. How could one survive such?"

Therefore, you should not move your eyes, your hands, or your feet haphazardly. You should depend on the soul to keep them. Those who are learning to nourish life often nurture their soul. They let their soul be the lord. If the lord does not leave, the residence will not collapse nor be destroyed.

THOSE WHO KNOW THE SPIRIT AND THE BREATH MAY LIVE LONG. THOSE WHO KEEP VOIDNESS AND NON-BEING WELL, NOURISH THE SPIRIT AND THE BREATH.

The Tao Book (TAO TE CHING) states, "My life depends on me. It does not depend on heaven and earth".

What is troubling regarding heaven and earth is that people do not know the supreme way (TAO.) For those who know about it but don't know how to practice it, they would live long, would they do the following only: they should clean out the mind. They should empty the mind, cut off anxiety, guard the breath and nourish the essence (or sperm.) Don't be bothered or involved by the circumstances of love and lust.

Lead a simple and plain life so that you can nourish the spirit and the breath. The way to longevity will thus be achieved.

IF THE SPIRIT IS CIRCULATING, THE BREATH IS CIRCULATING. IF THE SPIRIT STAYS STILL THEN THE BREATH REMAINS, TOO.

The so-called Yi (the mind) is the horse of the breath. When moving or stopping, they follow each other. If you do not want the Original Breath to leave the Hsüan-P'in, (the dark female) you should protect the supreme spirit. If the spirit does not leave the body, the breath stays, too. The breath will not be dispersed either. Naturally, you will be secure inside. You won't be hungry, nor thirsty.

IF ONE WANTS LONGEVITY, ONE SHOULD LET THE SPIRIT AND THE BREATH POUR INTO EACH OTHER.

What is this pouring into each other? It means that the spirit and the breath do not leave each other. Hsiun Gang said, "If even the least bit of the Yang breath remains, one cannot become a ghost. If just a tiny bit of the Yin breath is still there, one cannot become an immortal." The Original Breath is the Yang breath. What one takes in, is the Yin breath. If one lessens the intaking often and cuts down one's desires, one makes the Original Breath circulate inside the body. If the Original Breath is strong enough, the Yin breath will be lessened and naturally disappear. If the Yang is strong and the Yin is weak, hundreds of illnesses will be prevented from coming. The spirits are appeased and the body is (in a) pleasant (state.) One can hope for longevity.

IF A PERSON'S MIND IS NOT EXCITED WITH THOUGHTS, THERE IS NO COMING AND NO GOING, THERE IS NO EXITING AND NO ENTERING, THEN, (THE SPIRIT) CONSTANTLY ABIDES NATURALLY (INSIDE.)

Spirit and breath are originally one inside the mother's womb untill (the time) the baby is born. At the time it is born, (the baby) gets involved with the outside circumstances of love and lust, so that it cannot even for a short moment return to its original (state.) People know this and often cut off emotions and thought in order not to let the spirit leave. If one can remember this and practice it for a long time, the spirit will stay naturally inside the body.

PRACTICE THIS DILIGENTLY, IT IS THE REAL GENUINE WAY (TAO.)

The way of nourishing the genuine is entirely as stated here. The sayings of the wise men may not be sought after haphazardly. Whenever one practices the Embryonic Breath, one's joints will ease up and communicate. The hair will be abundant and long. The nose should inhale the breath subtly and lead it (with the mind) into the four limbs and the hundreds of pores. When exhaling, let it go with no commotion. Later the breath will keep coming. Guide it and do not exhale. I urge you to do this very slowly. It was said to guide it and not to exhale it. It is not to be guided just into the throat but it should be diffused very subtly, as if it were an internal breath. Also, don't let it leak out and dissipate.

THE MOTTO FOR THE EMBRYONIC BREATH: "THIRTY-SIX SWALLOWING START FROM ONE SWALLOWING. THE EXHALATION SHOULD BE REALLY FINE."

The inhalation should be extremely soft and continuous, whether sitting down or lying down. If you are walking or standing, you should be relaxed. What is forbidden is noise. Avoid anything that has a strong odor. It is called Embryonic Breathing, yet actually it is the internal elixir. It not only cures diseases, it also determinedly extends life. If one practices this long enough, one's name will be listed with the superior immortals.

The end of the TAI HSI CHING CHU.

COLOPHON

I examined the Yi-Wen-Lüeh which records the sections on Embryonic Breathing. It notes that there are thirty sections containing thirty-nine chapters. There are two chapters that are called "Treatise"; three, called "Technique"; sixteen, called "Oral Secrets". There is one each called "Essential", "Wonder", "Ode" or "Song". There are only three that are called "Ching". Originally, the author's name was unknown (to me) till I read Pao-P'u-Tzu's (book) which carries a chapter on the Embryonic Breathing. So I came to know that this book had been in circulation since the Tsin or Sung (dynasties, 317-477 A.D., N.T.) It still did not record that what had been authored by Huan-Chen was none other than this. But now, (I found this noted) in a Taoist book that I opened and copied it in my official residence so that it can be published. In the future, at my leisure, when I shall rest my mind in "the mysterious female" and swallow breaths for "the spirit of the valley", wouldn't I depend on this book?

Romances of Lo-Fu written at "the Residence of Mending the Natural Disposition."

T'AI HSI MI YAO KO CHÜEH
THE SECRET SONGS
ABOUT THE EMBRYONIC BREATH SECRET.

(Tao Tsang vol. IV. p.208. There are no separate section-numbers in the Harvard Yenching and the Wieger editions.)

BLOCKING THE BREATH.

If you suddenly have a disease that does not involve an injury, gather up your mind and go to a room where you can be at ease. Take off your clothes and lie down on your back on the bed and hold your fists tight. Tap your teeth (often) and burn incense. After you have swallowed 36 swallowings (and done the corresponding blockings) of the breath, the breath in the elixir field will exceed what is normally there. Use your mind to guide it to where you feel the ailment. That is the best way. When perspiration appears, it is the sign to stop. Do not do it in excess so you may reap the best benefits.

SPREADING THE BREATH.

The spreading of the breath is to be used to cure other people's illnesses as well.

If a person has been practicing the nourishing and the concentration of the essence for a long time, this person's body will have the Embryonic Breath. Whenever other people have any ailments and if the illness is known, the sick person should come to the person with the lord's breath, (that is the Embryonic Breath, N.T.) Cleanse your mind. Do not take it lightly. The person with the Embryonic Breath can transmit the genuine breath to help the sick person swallow it down. Have the sick person swallow in succession and use his mind to guide the breath where the ailment is. In a short while the ailment will disappear. The ghost or the evil will naturally escape. The (sick person) will be free from ailments.

THE SIX KINDS OF BREATHING.

(In the Preface to the second volume of THE PRIMORDIAL BREATH, the reader will find lengthy quotes on how the six exhalation sounds should be practiced. The subscripts indicate the pronouncing tone of each character. N. T.)

When practicing the six kinds of breathing, if you feel that there is a difference, then you should stop. Do not do it in excess. Your mind and breath would be damaged by overdoing it. The six kinds of breathing are as follows:

(1) The HSI_4. The HSI_4 method is the most magic and it should be kept (secret.) It belongs to the nose externally and internally to the lungs. If you feel cold, hot, tired, stuffy or have skin diseases you will surely get rid of such unpleasantness by using this kind of breathing.

(2) The HO_1. HO_1 belongs to the Ruler of the Heart. It rules the tongue. Whenever you feel the inside of your mouth is dry and rough, or you feel anxious or your body is hot, you should look at the degree of the ailment and use the HO_1 breathing to cure it. The lack of harmony of the cooking vessels and the viscera will naturally disappear.

(3) The HU_1. HU_1 belongs to the spleen. Its spirit rules the earth. If you are anxious, or stuffy or your abdomen is puffed up and your limbs are swollen, or if you have a

stuffiness that is hard to ease, use the HU_1 breathing to handle this. You will then be as good as before.

(4) The $HSÜ_1$. $HSÜ_1$ belongs to the liver. Its spirit rules the eyes. If you have red eyes and tears come down as if you are crying, it is all because the heat in your liver is rushing upward. Use the $HSÜ_1$ breathing to handle this. You will quickly or soon see the difference.

(5) The $CH'UI_1$. $CH'UI_1$ belongs to the kidneys. It rules the ears. If your loins, your waist or knees are often cold, or if the flow of the Yang (sperm N.T.) is stopped, you should subtly use the $CH'UI_1$ to handle this. Do not go outside and seek medicine.

(6) The HSI_1. HSI_1 belongs to the three cooking vessels. Whenever there is an ailment relating to the three cooking vessels, the three cooking vessels are injured by inharmonious breath. Just use the HSI_1 to handle this.

HARMONIZE THE SALIVA.

The lack of harmony usually comes from eating the 5 flavors. You have the three cooking vessels blocked and stuffed. You would feel heat and roughness, and sometimes you would feel coldness and plenty of puffing because of your body fluids. If you have these symptoms, you should use the Original Breath to cure it. Do not furthermore go to the kettle and ladle (meaning do not eat anymore, N.T.) If you feel hot, you should then rely on the HO_1 breathing (these exhalations are explained later in the text in more detail, N.T.). The heat will retreat naturally. If you feel coldness, it is proper to use the $CH'UI_1$ exhalation to make it disappear. In the meantime you should often rinse the inside of your mouth and swallow. The saliva will naturally be harmonious. The feeling of coldness or heat will stop if you do like this.

EAT AND DRINK WHAT IS PROPER.

If you would like to see the genuine goal of the nourishing way (TAO), you should choose what is proper by eating with refinement. For breakfast, plain rice gruel or plain rice cereal will make your thirst disappear. Sesame oil will moisten your throat and make your saliva adequate and abundant. The Non-glutinous rice is usually proper. Plain flour dough dumpling is also beneficial. Drinking good wine will usually make anger disappear. Hundreds of illnesses will stop if you take raw pepper. It is proper, before eating, to swallow six or seven swallowings of the breath. You should usually depend on eating. You should do the HO_1 breathing for three to five times after eating so as to prevent the poisonous breath from bothering the chest or the mind.

WHAT IS TO BE BANNED FROM EATING AND DRINKING.

You should go into a well secluded room without any opening or draft. The bed should be high enough to avoid the blowing of the ghosts. To be benefited you should hide the essence (not ejaculate sperm, N.T.) If you can keep the breath, your life will not be injured. Emotions of happiness or anger should be put away. Discourage your mind from pursuing profits and vanity. The genuine spirit and the real possessions should be guarded. Any poultry or fowl, beef in the form of paws, claws, head, limbs, any kinds of meat with blood (should be avoided.) You endanger your own life by eating these. Vegetables with pungent flavor or raw vegetables are bad for the breath. Whether you are hungry or not hungry, it is the same thing: you should avoid eating raw, hardened, or cold food. Sour food, salty food or acrid food is not proper. The clouds and the rain (sexual activity, N.T.) should stop. You should stop the thundering and the lightning (ejaculating, N.T.) especially in your late years. You should not take thick radish soup. A bowl of plain noodle soup will not harm you. Furthermore, you should avoid hot food.

Melons and fruits should not be abandoned. Stale food or food with foul smell is damaging. What is dead and raw, is dirty and not beneficial, you should not take such. Use breathing. Do not have doubts.

THE CUTTING OFF OF FOOD.

If you are persistent in your mind during thousands of days of exercising, the (three) corpses or the three worms will be naturally and gradually destroyed. The three elixir fields will be full and solid. You will have firm and strong bones and joints. You should think of cutting off reasons for eating. You should be lazy with tasting, eating or drinking. Whenever your stomach is empty, swallow (the breath) down to the navel. The Original Breath will take the place of the food which has been cut off. When you are full, your mind will be at peace and you should be diligently nurturing the inside. Whenever you are hungry, close (your mouth) and swallow. Do not speak, do not say any word. If you practice this way hard enough and long enough, the merit will be accomplished. Then you will believe that the nourishing of life depends on such secrets. It is not like the ordinary people's taking of medicine. You should practice all day long without any break. If you manage to take the medicine, its effect will only become void. It is difficult to persist in toiling with the tolerance of hunger. Only if you can constantly ingest the supreme harmonious essence (breath) can you have clean, clear brilliancy and pleasantness. If you are greedy of the outside beauty, this will interfere with the proper origin. Hundreds of diseases will assault your body and you will naturally become weak and (in) bad (shape.)

CAREFUL NURTURING.

You should very firmly and carefully nurture the essence (the sperm) and the breath, so that you may reap the benefits in your life and have longevity. A person with many desires and lusts will destroy his body. Those who would like to get rid of them can accomplish eternal life. If you worry about sickness before sickness appears, the sickness can not act. If you wait until calamities come, to get rid of them, this is hard to achieve. If you wait until you are upon your death bed to treasure your frail body, it will be too late, since the body has decayed already. Lusts and emotions, if not totally cut off, bring calamities, even if you are diligent in nourishing the Embryonic Breath. Only when one has the internal elixir, is the Way (TAO) completed. There are really few such people.

THE MERIT OF CHANGING IN NINE YEARS.

A person's breath, blood, veins, flesh, bone marrow, tendons, bones and hair are all formed in order. If you want to get rid of weakness and old age, of senility, and return to youth, you should undergo change every year for nine years. At first, you should sit properly and calm down. Close your eyes and stop breathing. Then sound the heavenly drum for 32 times. Use your tongue to lick the external part of your upper lip for nine times. Then lick the external part of your lower lip for nine times, and then, lick the inside of your upper lip for nine times. Then lick the inside of your lower lip for nine times. That is to say: the outer-upper lip is the southern direction; the lower outside lip is the northern direction; the inside of the upper lip is the eastern direction and the inside of the lower lip is the western direction, the tongue being at the center. Wait till your mouth is full of saliva, then puff up both cheeks several times. Inhale for twenty-one times. Subtly blow out a little from the nose. Then swallow. When you are swallowing, you should have a noise in the throat. It indicates that the saliva is coming down to the lower elixir field. Do it this way for three or five times, and note that when you are swallowing, you should wait till the breath has come out and then swallow.

The end of the T'AI HSI MI YAO KO CHÜEH.

T'AI CH'ING FU CH'I K'OU CHÜEH
THE EXTREMELY PURE
SECRET ORAL TRADITION OF
BREATH INGESTION
(Attributed to Kuo Chang)
(Tao Tsang, Vol. XXX, p.850; Harvard Yenching 569; Wieger 815)

The production of the thousands of beings and things depends on the Yin and Yang (forces.) They accomplish myriads of Yin and Yang transformations. They follow the Original Breath to separate cold from heat. Thus, (when) the Extreme Yang (the sun) prospers, warmth and various things are being produced. When the Extreme Yin (the moon) moves, the hoary air is destroying (all) kinds of sprouting. All (such) productions and destructions, though, do not happen without the influence of the Original Breath. This is familiar to the knowledgeable adept.

It was said, therefore, that heavens cannot slay and the earth may not hide those who eat the Original Breath, and this is excellent. Moreover, if you can connect the Original Breath between the kidneys and the nose, if you can spread the Yin and the Yang (forces) among the (five) viscera, then your in and out breathings will be unfailing and your practice of (inside) nourishing will be without perversity. You may expect to begin prolonging (your) life.

What I record here (on paper) is an oral secret, which is the method of ingesting the Original Breath. It has many secrets that are only taught orally, and it is impossible to record such with a brush on paper. What is here may be only a rough statement, yet it represents more or less the essential teaching of one sect. Should (these teachings) become available to someone interested in them, they should not be disclosed lightly.

In general, a human's abdomen has three divisions. One of the divisions is below the heart. If, as a beginner in the study of the art of breath ingestion you feel that the abdomen (division) below your heart is full, you should eat little. If you apply yourself to it for long, you will feel a natural communication downward, reaching the viscera.

Below the viscera, there is another division. If you feel that your abdomen is full, you should continue this practice for a long time. Then you will perceive (the breath) passing naturally below the navel into the TAN-T'IEN (the elixir field.) It may be observed then that a complete circulation of the breath occurs in the body, though it may not yet enter the "CHIU-CHUNG (lower abdomen, N.T.)" Later on, it will be observed that this gathered breath does exit from the "CHIU-CHUNG". Then, you can cure other people's illnesses.

When beginning such a study, you should pacify your body by abiding in quietude. You should practice constantly and carefully. If the breath enters the abdomen, then regardless whether you walk, stand, sit down, or lie down, it abides in all these situations and does not hinder the breath inside the abdomen. As long as the breath has not reached (the lower division), one cannot undertake the practice in all of these situations. The stabilizing work is difficult to achieve.

The beginning of the breath ingestion (practice) consists in inhaling breath. Stop the breath then for a little while, as if blocking it. When the breath is full and is to be exhaled, two thirds only may be exhaled. Then stop for a little while and swallow it. After swallowing, repeat (the procedure) until the abdomen is full. Then stop. It is necessary to do this in four different periods daily. Because for the beginning practitioner, breath has not yet entered the TAN-T'IEN (elixir field), it is still easily dissipated. You should have the breath (practice done in a) continuous and uninterrupted (way.) Once the breath enters the TAN-T'IEN, it will not dissipate even if you do not ingest it. The four times (indicated for practice) are the morning, the evening, at midnight and at noon. If you feel fullness by your heart, do not ingest breath but chew a little bit of KAN TS'AO (Chinese licorice) or KUEI (cinnamon.) The fullness will then disperse to the TAN-T'IEN. If you do not feel the fullness, then it is not full. When the Original Breath goes down, naturally you feel a little bit of stuffiness (in the chest.)

When starting, you must practice ingesting breath during the four periods (indicated.) In the morning and in the evening, use the postures of lying on the back and on the stomach, whereas at midnight and noon, use only the position of lying face up. When lying face up, you should use a low pillow and lie down on your back, pull both feet together, set your knees upright, extend both hands along your sides, and (only) then start swallowing breath. If you understand how to swallow properly, after merely ten swallowings the breath will fill the TAN-T'IEN (elixir field.) Wait then a short while after the swallowing is done. Use your will to escort the Breath to enter the "CHIU-CHUNG". When lying face down, the abdomen should lay bare against a warm bed; use some quilt to support the chest so it is propped up higher. Hands and feet should be extended and touching the bed. Swallow then ten swallowings. At each swallowing, use the will to convey the breath down the spine and then let it exit from the cooking viscera.

Each morning and evening, when ingesting breath, start first by lying face down and afterwards face up. Each swallowing of breath must be done in an audible manner. If you cannot make the swallowing audible, the work is in vain.

The swallowing of the breath must be done deep inside the throat, and slowly. You should not do it vehemently, for when done violently, coughing appears. Whenever swallowing breath, there should be a ten-breathing interval between each swallowing. It is like doing all other things. You must rest in order to be relaxed and comfortable.

Whenever you swallow breath, do not do it together with saliva. When swallowing the breath, you must do it in a dry way. If saliva appears in the swallowing, do not swallow it. When swallowing the saliva, you must inhale lest the raw air comes in. You must be extremely careful.

As you start receiving the method of breath ingestion, you need to chant the incantation. After you have received the method, when you are alone and proceding as usual, it is no longer necessary to chant the incantation. Should you, however, use (the method) to cure other people's sickness, then you have to chant the incantation every time.

In general, you may ingest the breath at other times than at the four (established) periods. Even when it is not at the right time, whenever you perceive little breath strength, or some weakness inside the stomach, you are to swallow your breath at will, regardless of whether it is much or little.

At the beginning of the ingesting (practice), the breath is not firm yet. Most of it will leak out and go down through the cooking viscera. You should solidify the breath so that this leakage should definitely not occur. Use your will to revolve the breath and disperse it down. When you begin ingesting breath, your thoughts and your will must be at peace. You should entertain no doubts, no fear, no worry and no apprehension. If you are fearful or apprehensive, it will then be difficult for the breath to circulate.

When ingesting breath, if you want your entire body to be in harmony, you should be of a complacent mind. There should be no interest in myriads of affairs. You will then improve day by day and be joyful and pleased without limit.

You should not think of eating when ingesting breath. You have to do it comfortably without any thoughts. Should you think of food, suppress such (thoughts) as if you did not even have any desire (to eat.) If you cannot suppress (such thoughts) in your mind, do the following: If thirsty, boil a soup made from the PI-LI (Ficus Pumila Linn.) with a little bit of fresh ginger. Bring to a boil once or twice. Drink one cup and your thirst will be quenched. A soup of ginger and honey will also do. If you are able to suppress the thoughts of eating, then even if faced with a feast all day long, you will not give a thought to it.

Just don't miss the proper (four) sessions for breath ingestion. If the TAN-T'IEN is constantly full and the breath is not allowed to exit for a whole day, even sexual activity will not hinder (the practice.) After having practiced ingesting for a long time and being accustomed to it, missing the proper session once or twice presents no harm.

The ingesting of breath with your face up is to clear out water, while doing it with your face down is to excrete food. The food (processing) viscera are on your right (side), the water (processing) viscera are on your left. After having ingested breath for a long time, breath will naturally get into the CHIU-T'OU, (the upper collector.) When lying face down and swallowing breath, concentrate (your mind) along your spine and then rest your thoughts and concentrate inside the abdomen. Try to listen to the noise going down close to the spine and then coming out from the cooking viscera. Listen to the noise and follow it as it goes down along the right side.

When swallowing breath, you cannot prevent it from leaking down if you are full and stuffy. It is not like what was described about protecting the breath and making it exit only from the top and the four limbs. If you practice this for long, you will spontaneously perceive (this happening.) But, even if you cannot observe it, you should rely only on this keeping of the breath. If you ingest breath for long, you have breath in the TAN-T'IEN (elixir field.) If you pat it and (hear) the sound "PENG PENG", then you must have done it right. Even if the heart (upper division) is not yet full, it is still all right. If you want the heart (upper division) to be full, you have to take in more breath, then you will have the breath as if by magic.

If you practice for long, you will naturally perceive it. There is no other method. You may ask, "How do I get it?" It is like eating and ingesting. You often take one step (at a time.) At the beginning of the study, it is reasonable to do like that. After a very long time, you can combine the eating and the ingesting into one. After the breath is ingested, it will circulate throughout the body. Do not force it to exit, but let it exit naturally.

If your strength for carrying out the daily business is weak, then you should swallow. You should not wait for the proper periods, or the time when you can internally see that the stool in your guts is exhausted. If you close your eyes and try to look internally, you will see that it is extremely hard to exhaust all the stool. Even if you cut off food, it takes more than twenty days to have it all exhausted. When you begin to cut off food, you must skip one or two meals daily for the first fourteen days. Just take boiled vegetables so as to help push out the stale stool. At each meal, it is not harmful to eat a bowl of MU-SU-CHIE (Medicago sativa) or WU-CHING (Brassica Rapa Depressa - raw turnip) and SUNG (Pinus Sinensis.) Boil off the bitter juice and put in a little bit of fat. Add some salt, bean sauce and vinegar to give it flavor according to taste. Don't add rice or noodles, etc. If you want to exhaust the breath of grains inside the intestines, you must eat vegetables. After four or five days, you should do away with the vegetables and drink only their juice. Then, after about three more days, stop totally. You must drink a little wine. Empty the inside of your stomach according to the natural disposition. After that, drink a larger amount so as to vomit any phlegm from inside the chest. It is extremely good to eat pepper two or three times every day. Select from one tenth of a pint of pepper the grains that have no seeds and the closed ones and remove any dirt. Use wine, water, PI-LI (Ficus Pumila Linn.) soup or vegetable juice to swallow the pepper (grains) down. It benefits the breath and pushes down bad substances from inside the stomach. This is the secret method. The ginger's nature is to be able to break down substances. If there is food inside the stomach, it is all right to take the ginger soup, but if the food is all exhausted, then it is not proper.

If among the vegetables there is some HSIEH-HAO, (Seseli Libanotis var. Daucifolia) and cilantro, you must not take ginger soup since it is capable of upsetting the breath. In general, if you lie face up when swallowing, then the breath enters the guts and is transported into the CHIU-CHUNG. If you lie face down when swallowing, you should transport (the breath) to have it exit from the cooking viscera. Human beings have cooking viscera and raw viscera. If you practice for one month, the breath begins to enter the coiled intestines and makes a small sound when revolving and circulating through the guts. This is the right method. In general, it is superior for a human being to have a great number of coils to his intestines. To have under twelve coils, maybe ten, nine, possibly seven, five or three, is inferior. People of low station have big and short intestines. Those people can listen but they do not have any wisdom. When a person's intestines are big, he is able to listen. When a person's intestines are short, he is without any wisdom. It is desirable and superior to have long intestines. If the intestines are short and small, they do not belong to humans. The mind causes a divine breath. The liver causes an enduring breath. The lungs are (actually) killing the breath, the spleen causes the TAO breath. The kidneys cause the Original Breath. What is correct to swallow is the internal breath.

In general, if a man's intestines are long, breath is easy to solidify, whereas if they are short, breath is hard to solidify. When ingesting breath, and when the revolving has been stirred up inside the intestines, and there is noise, then lie on your bed on your right side and use your right hand to support your head. Use your left hand to pull your left leg and to bend it. Straighten up your body and your right leg. Swallow the breath and (imagine that) it enters your right leg. And that's it. After a long practice, the breath makes a sound each time it goes down. The sound turns along the coiled intestines. It yields and makes a sound. You should remember to count the coils. If the sound of flowing and revolving is the soft YU, YU sound, then this is a good flow and circulation. Human intestines have four main coils. They have sections and pits. You should also count and record for yourself the number of such sections and pits.

THE SECRET OF THE DISTINCTION BETWEEN THE OUTSIDE BREATH AND THE ORIGINAL BREATH

The Original Breath and the outside breath should not be mixed. If the raw breath is swallowed and enters, it must be let out from below to get rid of it. It must not stay inside the intestine. If the circulation of the breath is proper and responds to the brain, warm breath will ascend to the brain. The breath may descend towards the feet in the same manner.

If the Yang breath is revolving first, then you start by perceiving cold first and then heat in your feet. Why is it like this? It is because the Yang breath pushes out the Yin breath. This is why it is like this. (On the other hand), if the Yin breath is revolving first, then the Yang breath exits first and your feet are first very hot and afterward they begin to cool off. All other organs behave the same. If you are able to revolve the breath so as to enter your head, it removes wrinkles from your face.

(There is apparently a break in the text here, N.T.)

What follows is FROM THE LAO CHÜN T'AI HSÜ T'AI SHANG WU SHANG TZU JAN T'AI CH'I BOOK (THE BOOK OF THE SAGE LAO ENTITLED: THE EXTREMELY GREATLY ELEVATED VOID, THE UNSURPASSED, NATURAL GREAT BEGINNING.)

In Lao (Tzu's) method of managing the body and keeping the One, when the Original Breath begins to be produced at midnight, you must sweep your teeth with your tongue and lick your upper and lower lips. Use your nose to inhale the breath and your mouth to swallow it twenty-seven times, then stop. The live breath circulates and flows inside the hundred arteries. It brings about man's longevity.

Lao (Tzu's) method to manage the body (is as follows): Rise up in the morning. First exhale into both palms with the $Hsü_1$ (sound) and rub them till they heat up. Spread the heat evenly onto your forehead fourteen times. This is called "To protect the NI-WAN (MUD PILL)"; it equips the human body with spirits.

Next in managing the body, rub both hands till you make them warm and rub your face fourteen times. This is called "the dry bathing"; it gets rid of the evil breath. The face is the one-foot (tall) dwelling in which a genuine man abides. If you see this man, you will not be sick. Next, rub both hands again till they are warm, spread the warmth evenly throughout your trunk fourteen times. This is called "the washing of the body"; it enables you to get rid of cold winds.

Next rub (again) both hands till they become warm and from the forehead, spread the warmth evenly to the hair on your head fourteen times in order to nurture and keep the soul of your hair alive. It is called "to wash the head" It enables the human hair not to turn white and the teeth to grow again, if they fall out. Next, rub both hands till they become hot and fork your fingers upward from below your ears through both ears fourteen times. It makes the hearing to be acute. Each ear has respectively two spirits. (Both) spirits' names are "CHIAO-NÜ" (the graceful ladies.)

The method to manage the body and keep the One is for you to rise up in the morning and after having gotten dressed, to have your hands touch your head while chanting the (following) incantation: "It is a great luck to prolong life and remove hundreds of diseases and reach the door of happiness. The five viscera are harmonized, entirely free of worries and calamity. All the spirits abstain themselves and follow me to help me reach old age without being afraid of anyone."

After finishing the incantation, when getting up, first step out with your left foot and chant CH'IEN ("HEAVEN".) Next, step out with your right foot and say the incantation: "YUAN" ("ORIGINAL".) Next, step out with your left foot and again chant "HENG" ("SUCCESS".) Next, step out with your right foot and chant: "LI" ("PROFIT".) Next, step out with your left foot and chant "CHEN CHI" ("VIRTUOUS LUCK".) This is the same as saying, "Heavenly, Original, Success and Profit are (but) names for the virtuous body which is lord over the ten thousand spirits. When the jade doors (the eyes) see the white sun, it is a great luck and a realization of expectations."

The method to keep the One is to cherish the breath constantly and to be sparing of words. This means to make breath enter in large amounts but let it come out only a little. Use the breath to nurture the Original. Think of the Original Breath and (you will) eventually succeed in prolonging your life.

The method of keeping the One is to lie down often, according to the four periods and the eight yearly terms CH'UN (beginning of spring around February 5-18), 2. LI-HSIA (beginning of summer around May 5-18), 3. LI-CH'IU (beginning of autumn around August 7-21), 4. LI-TUNG (beginning of winter around November 7-21), 5. CH'UN-FEN (the vernal equinox), 6. CH'IU-FEN (the autumnal equinox), 7. HSIA-CHIH (the summer solstice), 8. TUNG-CHIH (the winter solstice.) In the spring and summer, rise early with the rooster. In autumn and winter, rise late, waiting first for the sun to appear without getting bored (waiting.) To do otherwise means to harm yourself

A PRAYER FOR THE BODY

"Carefully I present my body with the five viscera, the six receptacles, the nine palaces, the twelve divine rooms, the four limbs, the five parts, the tendons, the bones, the marrow, the brain, the skin, the blood arteries, the cavities and openings, the blood, the breath, one hundred eighty muscle passes, the three hundred sixty bone joints, the one thousand two hundred form shadows, and the twelve thousand brilliant essences. On the left, there are three (upper) souls (HUN), and on the right, seven (lower) souls (P'O.) As for the three ghosts and five spirits, they wear the vermilion bird (hat) on their head, and the black warrior (shoes) on their feet. On the left, the green dragon is supported, while on the right, the white tiger is held. To support the green dragon means to welcome. To hold the white tiger means escorting off. The vermilion bird leads in front with a flag. The black warrior follows in the rear with a cup and a drum. All these enable my heart not to suffer from evil, my liver not to suffer from pain, my lungs not to suffer from debauchery, my kidneys not to suffer from weariness, my spleen not to undergo death, my gall not to suffer from fright, and my stomach not to suffer from uncleanness. My excited breath is all the more eager to do the breathing exercises as I have proclaimed."

If you walked in the dirt and are in a state of uncleanness, then bathe, wash yourself and rinse your mouth off to free the form from dirtiness. The method is to use ten ounces of bamboo leaves, four ounces of the white meat of peaches that have been peeled off. Use twelve pecks (about 13.5 gallons) of clean water to boil all this once, let it cool off to a comfortable temperature in order to use it for bathing. Ten thousand sicknesses will be removed. For a bather, this boiled water is not only to boil off the (three) dirty corpses, it can also be used for bathing. If so, do not wash your head with it. Then, proceed with bathing according to the ordinary bathing method.

The end of the T'AI CH'ING FU CH'I K'OU CHÜEH

T'AI CH'ING T'IAO CH'I CHING
THE BOOK ON THE EXTREMELY PURE HARMONIZING OF THE BREATH
(attributed to Ko Hsien Kung)
(Tao Tsang Vol. XXX, p.834; Harvard Yenching 569; Wieger 813)

(INTRODUCTION)

A book[1] on immortality states, "At midnight, at the TZU hour (11 pm-1 am) swallow 9x9 or 81 (times); when the cock crows, (swallow) 8 x 8 or 64 (times); at day break, (swallow) 6 x 6 or 36 (times); at breakfast time, (swallow) 5 x 5 or 25; (times); between 9-11 am., (swallow) 4 x 4 or 16 (times.)"

The method (described) above is worldly (vulgar, nothing more than an) old book handing down a teaching of erroneous action. (Though) practicing swallowing for long, it

---

[1] It refers probably to the fourth book or section of Chih Yen Tsung (A Summary of the Best Sayings) to be found in the Tao Tsang Vol. XXXVIII, p.569.

will waste away in vain years and months, (showing nothing but) a toilsome and difficult progress, the verification of which will not be achieved to lengthen (life), but, on the contrary, it will injure (it.)

There are many people like that who do not (know how to) swallow the Original Breath and do not recognize (its) arcane root. Consequently, (they) swallow for a long time without any effect. (Their) souls decline, their breath withers within. (These are) people who admire the TAO in vain and injure (their) lives. How pitiful! Certainly it is not the correct secret of the way (TAO.) It is not to be relied upon in practice.

Also, (such) old books speak of ceasing all at once with (eating) cereals, and of a method to swallow the breath day and night, totaling 540 swallowings during the twelve periods. When the twelve periods have passed, (one) has to start all over again. If a man, who is in his prime, wastes (himself) violently in profits and desires and is ignorant of the correct breath, how could (he even) think to perfect and nourish his body, rest his ambition, and quiet his soul? When he approaches old age, the five viscera have (actually) been injured. If he suddenly interrupts food (fasts) without a gradual progress in nourishing and repairing (his body), then the Original Breath is not yet up to standard and the common food has been cut out. Thus both (breath and food) are interrupted. That leads to danger and death. His desire to perfect his body cannot be attained.

(The book) states also (falsely N.T.) that the limit for swallowing is a great amount and the fullness is the merit result (to be looked for.) (But) a man who begins to swallow breath within (the first) 100 days has hardly any communication and circulation (of the breath.) The previously (blocked) joints do begin to open up. But to begin suddenly to swallow so as to cause fullness of breath will render the stomach sick with swelling and stuffiness. (This is) absolutely not the correct TAO (principle.)

Correspondingly, start with swallowing little. After three years, one may do as one wishes, swallowing a lot. However, for a beginner, his limb joints are not opened up and his muscles and skin are also still closed. If he then suddenly undertakes much swallowing (of the breath), it will result in the stomach becoming swollen and stuffy. How could one succeed?

(The same book) states also (falsely N.T.) that before noon the breath is alive, while after mid-day (the breath is called) "death breath." According to this book the live breath may be swallowed (while) the death breath should not be swallowed. What kind of saying is that?

Though man (should) eat three times each day, sometimes, because of travel or perhaps pressing business, the proper time (to eat) is missed. If one happens upon food, one just eats. Why should one wait for a proper time? Breathing is similar. When there is breath, swallow it without giving thought whether the breath is of the live or dead (type.)

It also (falsely, N.T.) states, "(Take) a long inhalation through the nose to fill the mouth with air, then swallow it. Afterwards, exhale only a little bit, but inhale a lot."

The TAO (principle) of breath swallowing at its root is called the Embryonic Breath. This Embryonic Breath is like a baby in the mother's womb. During ten months, though it does not eat, it is able to grow, to form (its) thin bones and tender muscles. The reason why it is able to tighten the fists and guard the One is that it has no thought except the Original Breath. The moment it exits the mother's womb, it inhales the outside air, gives a cry, knows dryness and dampness, hunger or satisfaction, and it loses the Original Breath. At present, (what) the nose inhales and is swallowed is on the outside and (actually) should not be taken to be swallowed.

(The above mentioned book) also states: "Obtain the live breath of the five directions with the mind facing toward the particular direction and thinking thoughts. Begin (by thinking to obtain) the green breath of the East; next, the red breath of the South; next the white breath of the West, and then the black breath of the North and the yellow breath of the center. In everything (one must) think of the five directions and the (corresponding) breath color to swallow it."

In short, (all of the above) is incorrect. First of all this swallowing of breath has to be done without thinking. Consequently, the harmonious breaths will come naturally. Then, when swallowing them, each (breath) will return to its (proper) place and not one will be misplaced. Moreover, the five directions are each in the five viscera, so what is there to think about? To have thinking is to cause an arising of production of destiny. Consequently, the mind is unsettled. If the mind is unsettled, then the breath is not quieted. If the breath is not quieted, then it is unnatural. If unnatural, then the breath loses its rhythm and then bad breath is inhaled. When inhaling bad breath, suffering is then being produced. If suffering is produced, then the hundred illnesses are pouring in.

The Yellow Court Canon says, therefore, "Think inexhaustibly only of the one goal which is to prolong life. (All the spirits) do not reside separately but dwell entirely in the center of the brain. They position themselves in order, with their faces outward. What is to be guarded is (nothing but) the mind. Then everything will naturally be proper." It means what was discussed already. One's thinking of the five directions is not the right (way) to swallow.

The book also (falsely N.T.) states, "Swallow abundantly. (After) one hundred swallowings-in, the P'ENG sound is made. Therefore this is the wonder."

In general, in the beginning, the swallowing of breath has to be little to open up thoroughly, which means that the hundreds of hair pores will open up. Every closing of breath would cause sweating of the whole body. Even if you swallow suddenly one thousand breaths, there is no blocking. The "P'ENG, P'ENG" sound is still the non-communicating and blocking type. (Such a blocking of the breath) will turn a man's face yellow. It will injure the five viscera and his mind will be lost.

(The book) states also that while (one's sweat) during the first fifteen days exits from the hands, it exits afterwards from the feet.

Thinking should be exercised for use against occasional sickness. But if there is no sickness, it is not proper to incline to have thoughts. Therefore the Yellow Court Canon says: "If things do not offend each other, then the world is peaceful." It means (to have) no thinking.

(The book) also states, "When starting the swallowing of breath (practice), one should desire to desist from (eating) cereals. After the full twenty-one days, one is immune from hunger. Block the breath for ninety breaths, then swallow once so that the stomach is half full, and don't exhale much. The thought of non-attachment should communicate from the hair above to the feet below." (The book) further states: "Think (from) the feet upwards, along the kidneys to the throat, then again think of the five colored breaths and block them"

For the beginner to cut out (cereals) all of a sudden, as I have explained previously, it is wrong. To cut all of a sudden the five viscera (off cereals) will injure man. How could one be able to accomplish the exercises and be free from hunger after (only) 21 days? If the exercises (have been undertaken) for three years, the Original Breath is achieved. Consequently, it dwells in the sea of breath (the lower TAN T'IEN, N.T.) and coagulates (there.) Then, when one must interrupt the eating of (cereals), these will be interrupted (naturally.) Why (make) a principle of limiting it to a number of days, or even start to think (of such)?

(The book) states, "(During) ten breaths, bend a finger (to count) each breath. If (one) has reached a group of seventeen breaths, then swallow once. Perhaps (one may) stop the breath after four times nine, or after three hundred and sixty breathings. Then turn on the other side (to mark such.)"

When swallowing the correct breath, (one should) interrupt thinking, get rid of thought and guard the mind in the state of non-action (WU WEI.) (One should) abandon form into a body of non-action (WU WEI.) How could one bend fingers in order to keep count? Regardless of walking, standing, sitting down, or lying down, just let it come naturally. An empty stomach is convenient, so just swallow. Why tire oneself to turn from one side to another to keep track of the count?

(The book) states, "If there is no saliva juice in the mouth, then use one or two (Chinese) dates (ZIZYPHUS VULGARIS); eat the flesh, but keep the kernel (in the mouth) to induce saliva."

A beginner with no skill cannot have real (natural) saliva. The little saliva induced in this way is still unusable because it is not the real (natural) saliva.

It is said, also, to inhale long through the nose and swallow the breath when it is pressing. One should swallow it for long and in succession, just like water poured from a bottle. Doing it this way is practically killing a man. How could (such a practice) perfect the soul?

It is also written that by simply closing the breath, one can naturally have plenty of breath and be filled with it. This is enough (advice) to kill a person! It states, moreover, that in case of sickness, fight it by closing the breath and use (the different) exhalations corresponding to the five viscera (against the illness.)

If there is sickness which should be fought, one still does not know how to attack it, or whether to attack it a little or much. If one does not understand the proper timing and uses the breath to attack the sickness, it is again just a way to kill a person.

It is also said that the breath must be solidified and not let out below; it should be solidified and then be spread by exercising one's will.

What kind of sayings are these? The upper (part) of a human (body) has seven openings and there are two openings below. If the upper cooking vessel does not (freely) communicate and it has chills and fevers, it is because the breath is not harmonious among the three cooking vessels to prevent sickness.

If (one were) to begin to attack the (sickness), first (one's) breath would have to flow (properly) and be let out. If one, swallows (breath) above, it would (perforce) have to leak out below. Thus one must not solidify it. This will be explained later on, in detail.

THE METHOD OF SWALLOWING THE BREATH

In general (in order) to swallow breath, one must discern the proper timing of the breath and the (different) symptoms (of any) illness. While the entering breath (inhalation) is of (only) one (kind), the exiting breath (exhalation) is of six (kinds.) One should know the six (types) of exhalation and (only) then ingest (breath.)

Although the old books all talked about the shape of the mouth for the six exhalations, one only heard of the ways of how to detect their proper timing instead of how to recognize them. Now it is all recorded as follows:

If the reason why you want to learn the ingesting of breath is because the three cooking vessels are not communicating, swallow breath, but, do not let it stay in the upper vessel, because it may cause a stuffy chest (in which the breath) does not flow. You should learn first how to manage breath and to recognize the six (kinds) of exhalation in order to remove the bad air of the five viscera. Then you may swallow the breath. Then, the clean breath descends, and each swallowing will be beneficial.

In order to harmonize the breath, you must rely on the (existing) "door and window". By relying on the "door and the window" (is meant) the nose as the door of heaven, and the mouth as the window of the earth. It follows, then normally that the nose inhales and the mouth (should) exhale, and (this is) beneficial to breathing. If breath is inhaled with the mouth or exhaled through the nose, (this is) harmful to breathing. If it is harmful to breathing then (there is) obstruction. If it benefits breathing, then the breath circulates freely. It is because the Yin and Yang are used as the distinguishing principle. Now that you know of the door and the window, of what is harmful and beneficial, of the Yin and Yang as the distinguishing principle, you should rely on this nourishing practice.

Regardless whether you walk, stand, sit or lie down, the nose should ordinarily (be the one to) inhale and the mouth should be used ordinarily for exhalation.

The inhalation inhales the pure (air) and the exhalation exhales what is dirty. There is dirty (air) because it exits from the five viscera. Why do the five viscera have dirty air? On account of eating the five flavors, (each of) the five flavors (corresponds) to one of the five viscera. The turbid breath of each viscera is all exhaled through the same mouth.

Moreover, the breaths that are in the six receptacles collect at the same exit. They all thrust forward, combine, and become turbid breath. How can you find out about this turbid breath? During sleep at night, the mouth is generally closed; then the breaths of the five viscera are blocked in the throat from exiting. Every time upon awakening open your mouth and perceive it deliberately. There is a terribly dirty breath unbearable to the smell. You will, therefore, know this breath as being dirty and evil.

When the inside of the mouth is dry and the inside skin of the jaws feels rough, without saliva juice, and maybe the throat is hurting and one is unable to eat, this is the symptom of heat. Then, open widely your mouth and exhale with the HO_1 breathing.

At each HO_1 breathing, rely on the "door" and the "window" to do the breathing. After doing the HO_1 breathing ten or twenty times, sound the heavenly drum. This means tap (the upper and lower) teeth (together.) Tap the teeth together fifty-six times. Use the tongue to rinse the flowery pond and swallow the saliva juice. The Yellow Court Canon says, "Rinse and swallow the magic juice and calamities will not invade." This is what it means.

Also pant accordingly, letting breath enter and exit naturally to harmonize it. Do it three or more times. Then again open your mouth and do a big HO_1 breathing, harmonize it again. After doing it this way and becoming aware that the feverish breath has receded entirely, then stop. How can you know it? When the thick sweet clear water (saliva) inside the throat is produced, it is that the feverish breath has receded and the five viscera are cool. The Yellow Court Canon says, "Pour the clear water of the Jade Pond upon the magic root. (One) is able to nourish it carefully and can prolong one's existence." The pure thick sweet water is right here. If (one) is able constantly to harmonize and investigate like this, it is to be expected that the five viscera will never produce any sickness. If able to examine (what) is offered here, it is expected that the three cooking vessels will be able to communicate naturally, and then every swallowing of breath will be beneficial and the exercise is not in vain.

Breath is ruled by the mind. If the mind is unruly; then breath is unruly. If the mind is proper, then breath is proper. What raises the hands, moves the feet, and causes joy, anger, sadness or happiness - is all of the mind. The movement of the mind or thinking is certainly breath. Breath perceives the will. The will follows the mind. If breath is being perfected, then the body is perfected. If breath is interrupted, the soul gives up. If the soul is extinguished, then the body dies. The reason, therefore, why a doctor must first examine the pulse, is because within the five viscera in the four (different) seasons, the pulse is combined with the condition of the breath. (The doctor) investigates the source of the sickness and then finds out the (type of) medicine needed. If one would only find out the condition of (one's) breath, (one) could expect the five viscera to be naturally harmonious; and if the pulse is harmonious, the breathing would be comfortable. How can you know (this)? The five viscera are ruled by the five breaths and also by the five directions. If the viscera and the breath are harmonized, then the four seasons are favorable. Also, if one is able to observe naturally (the use of) the mouth and the nose, and the timing of the give and take, heat or cold can no more enter (the body) then.

The (aforementioned) book also talks about how to know of the heat and the cold.

There is only one entering breath while the exiting breath is of six kinds. These six kinds (of exhalations) are the HSI_4, the HO_1, the HU_1, the $HSÜ_1$, the $CH'UI_1$, and the HSI_1 exhalations. Five of the six breaths rule the five viscera respectively. The extra breath (or the sixth) belongs to the three cooking vessels.

The HSI$_4$ (breath) corresponds to the lungs. The lungs rule the nose. If the nose is cold or hot or inharmonious, rely on the HSI$_4$ breathing to regulate it. Moreover, if the skin has boils or bruises, rely on the HSI$_4$ (breathing) manner to regulate such.

The HO$_1$ (breath) corresponds to the heart and rules the tongue. If it is dry or rough and breath does not circulate, it is because of heat. Use the HO$_1$ (breathing) to get rid of it. If there is a great deal of heat, open the mouth widely. You must work with the will in the proper measure since any excess could injure you.

The HU$_1$ (breath) corresponds to the spleen, which rules the territory of the central palace (the abdomen, between the heart and the diaphragm.) If the breath is slightly hot and lacking harmony, if the stomach is puffy with full, stuffy air, and is not circulating or leaking, then use the HU$_1$ to regulate it.

The HSÜ$_1$ (breath) corresponds to the liver. The liver rules the eyes. If the eyes are feverish, one is able to use the HSÜ$_1$ breath to harmonize and regulate them.

The CH'UI$_1$ (breath) corresponds to the kidneys. The kidneys rule the ears. If the loins, the feet soles are cold and the sexual organs are weak, it is the CH'UI$_1$ (breath) that trains and regulates them.

The HSI$_1$ (breath) corresponds to the three cooking vessels.

In general, the afore-mentioned breaths belong for the most part, to the five viscera and the six receptacles and the three cooking vessels. Yet, unharmonized cold or heat is all connected to the heart.

The heart is ruled with the HO$_1$ (breathing.) Use only the HO$_1$ breathing to regulate (all of them.) Thousands of sicknesses are healed (by it.) Thus, one does not need to employ each and every one of the six kinds of exhalations to harmonize or (cure) sicknesses.

As soon as (you) rely too much, when training the breath, on breathing through the "door" (nose) and the "window" (mouth) then you may become aware of dryness inside the throat. If perceiving (such) dryness, close the mouth and use exclusively the nose for breathing. Juice will be produced inside the mouth and the inside of the throat will be moistened. Rinse (it) in order to be able to swallow it. Also, pay attention to the inside of the mouth. If it is free of heat and the turbid breath, the five viscera are harmonious. At that point, one does not need to train the (breath.)

Regardless of walking, standing, sitting or lying down, press the tongue to swallow the breaths. The color of the face will be bright.

The old book states also to try doing (the swallowing) in the Tzu period (11 pm - 1 am), when the ruling breath is produced, and to do it, also, in the six other periods at the proper time for ingesting and counting it.

Most of the beginners in the ingesting of the (breath) feel extremely hot, and most of them do not know how to proceed in the proper order or pace, to be gradually nourished. What can not be understood is that most people use only a (rigid) formula but have not actually sought to use the teacher's secret genuine method, and so, when the time comes to swallowing (breath), many (end up) injuring (themselves.) Sickness may be caused, or they may harm their chances of (living) to an old age. The number of such examples is really great.

Some said that there is no merit to (this art of) breathing; some said that the practice is completely without benefit. As years and months go by, what is the accomplishment within the time period? Maybe a person does not encounter a master to nourish his mind. Therefore, at the time when he is to remove the two doubts, his life is already mismanaged.

I will now somewhat reveal the merit of this science. I have studied and practiced both principles of what is injurious and what is beneficial. All this was transmitted (by me) in the great many years of my life. The genuine and the false have been seen altogether. From now on, practitioners will make no error and will gain more benefit daily. It will heal sickness like through magic and (the practice) has instant verification. (What) is good or bad will be immediately manifested.

In all the people who are beginners in this art, the three cooking vessels have not yet been opened up. All the ingested breath stays in the upper vessel. It does not pass from the upper cooking vessel. The breath dwells (there.) There is stuffiness in the breast, and if there is pressure (there), it might injure the practitioner. He who does not understand the principle of training must especially pay attention to it. The one beginning to swallow breath must first eat at proper times, because eating will turn against the proper order of the nourishing practice. One should be sincere and should not desist in getting rid of the Three Corpses. One should part with splendor and abandon nobility. One should be moderate in sex, and distance oneself from wealth. In this way, one begins to approach the TAO, and progresses daily. The practice of lengthening life is for sure not in vain. But should one be unable to practice according to this way, even if one knows it, one will accomplish nothing.

People who nourish the genuine are of three categories. The characteristics of the principles obtained are not uniform. One should not hold to them too rigidly. They are slightly elaborated herewith as follows:

The original disposition of the scholar of superior quality is reserved and leisurely. His thoughts are pure and elegant. (His) speech agrees with the TAO and his behavior is flawless. Such a man has these natural gifts from a previous life. It is like casting a stone into water. There is no comparison. These are the people with superior intelligence, and they manifest (their) heart's (intent) early.

The man of average quality may be personally maintaining (himself) in a splendid (social) status. Maybe (his) power and his reputation are high and lofty. Perhaps he has a powerful career and a wealthy marriage. Perhaps he has fame and a high position. Yet he is in doubt whether to advance further or to withdraw, and suddenly he may be injured. When hearing of the TAO, he will be disquieted all the time. Then, during a whole morning (he) cannot rest but think. His two thoughts are at war. If ever victorious, through this whole hesitation, he loses sixty or seventy percent (in prolonging life.) This illustration shows an average intelligence whose mind manifests itself late.

The scholar of inferior quality (allows) the two periods (youth and middle age, N.T.) to pass and is wasting his late years. The power of his muscles has decreased and is minimal, his mind and his soul are dying. Though he has emoluments, it is like dressing in brocade, yet walking in the night (nobody sees it, N.T.) He is like the sun setting in the West or a candle in the wind. (For him), finding his soul and thinking of the TAO is like biting his own navel (an unreachable goal, N.T.) If one thinks about this quietly, there is no end to the sighing (of sadness.)

If this group (of people described above) are able to concentrate the mind and encourage the will, ten or twenty percent can be saved. (If they are) eighty (years old) and above, the damage is already spread and settled. One can only pray for (their) next life. These are the three grades of humans.

The former sages abandoned their lament. Future generations should be careful. They should manifest their will from the deep root, and persist. Then they will be successful without failure. Their happiness and long life will be limitless. How could it be anything but ideal?

The ingestion of breath is originally called the Embryonic Breath. The Embryonic Breath is like a baby in a mother's womb. In ten months, though not eating (on its own), it is still able to develop, to be nourished and grow fine bones and soft sinews. It keeps its fists tightly closed and guards the One since it has received the correct breath from the beginning. It has neither thoughts nor worries. It is being completed, innocently receiving the Original Breath, accomplishing its metamorphosis, and opening its joints and viscera. All this happens by itself. Immediately upon exiting the womb and inhaling the outside breath as he is giving out (its first) cry, it experiences dryness, wetness and hunger. It seems that it has worries, then, it loses the Original Breath.

Now a practitioner's ingestion (of breath) is like a child in a mother's womb. What is called Embryonic Breath is (actually) the ingestion of the inner breath. (But when) the old book says, "Take in the outside breath through the nose and ingest it", this is surely not the correct method.

When (you want) to ingest breath, (you should) try at midnight after awakening from sleep, or after waking up in the fifth watch (3-5 AM) to harmonize breath as indicated before. Examine it properly. Rinse (the mouth) and swallow the magic juice (the saliva.) Then lie down face up, spread the hands and put a pillow under the feet. Then rest the mind, settling it into voidness, and cut off (any) thought. Breathe at will, relying on the "door" and the "window". Then breathe in and out quickly and close firmly the mouth. When there is internal breath (inside the lungs) make it go up to the mouth. Slightly puff up the mouth and swallow (the breath) down. As before, use the will to guide it (down and) use your hand to massage (your abdomen) to make the breath go down from the heart. Attend to harmonizing the breath six or seven times. Then swallow one breath and use your hands to massage as previously. After (you) have swallowed twenty breaths, stop. During daytime, attend to (it) any time at will, whether sitting, or lying down, whenever it is convenient, in quietude and security. Attend to swallowing more than ten swallowings. Each swallowing is to be separated by having harmonized the breath 40 or 50 times (in between.) Swallow very slowly. And if (you are) not busy, all the swallowings should not be done at the same time. With each swallowing, use your hands to massage your abdomen to bring (the breath) down, and use the will to escort it downwards; pay attention to it. If the upper cooking vessel does communicate, the swallowing goes deep down past the navel. When it does not communicate and it stays inside the breast, wait till meal time when you observe that the upper part (of the stomach) is empty and the breath flows below, communicating. Then eat at will. When you are not hungry, do not eat.

If eating, do not eat to the full, since, if you are full, this hinders the ingestion of breath. After having eaten and after (the spaces) above the heart and inside the stomach are slightly empty, then attend to ingesting less than twenty swallowings. Also, after the dinner time, when (the space) above the heart is empty, ingest twenty more swallowings (of breath) and then stop. Regardless of whether you are walking, standing, sitting, or lying down, have the same timing of ingestion as you had the previous day.

Do the same for one hundred days. For each ingestion (of breath), remember to massage (your abdomen) with your hands to disperse it. Each swallowing is better if separated by ten breathings or less. In the beginning of the ingestion of (breath), since the three cooking vessels do not communicate and the joints are not open, you should be careful not to block (the breath), and you should not do much ingesting (of breath.) Increase by 3-5 more swallowings every ten days, up to the time when the first hundred days have passed. After one hundred and fifty days, add four or five swallowings (per day) till (you) complete two hundred swallowings (per day.) In a year's time, breath circulates completely: joints open up, skin and flesh are nourished, hair pores open up (as well.) Just wait for the stomach to be empty, then swallow at will 3-5 times. Consecutively, swallow it (thus no more separately, N.T.) without restriction as (was done) before, but do not overdo it. (Stay) at three hundred swallowings (per day.) After three years, the breath does revolve completely and circulates greatly, the five viscera achieve (proper nourishment), the bones and marrow are strong and benefited, the skin is filled and solid. Then there is no limit to the number of swallowings (per day.) If one should interrupt (eating) cereals, one may do it now. But (if he were) to do it before (the first) three years, he would first suffer the five diseases (of the five viscera, N.T.) and then the seven injuries (of the five viscera, the body and the will, N.T.), the viscera and the receptacles would be injured, the hundred passes would wither away. If you are unable to progress gradually and try to interrupt suddenly the eating of meals to receive the benefit (of long life) or if in addition, (you are) not able to interrupt the thought of the worldly mind and constantly scheme for wealth and sex according to natural tendencies, and, if as usual, (you) would know a stomach only hungry for cereals and gradually fast yet not supplement with medicine, then new sickness would be produced and thousands of diseases would follow. How could you not die by just thinking and wanting (such)?

Moreover, after ingesting breath, you should know the order of eating. At breakfast, eat daily a little flavorless porridge. It harmonizes the spleen breath, (giving thus) the whole day enough saliva juice. At lunch eat one or two flavorless dough biscuits. You may also cook an onion or shallot broth. However, do not eat them hot. If you are hungry at dinner, eat a few flavorless hard flour dough dumplings. Boil them twenty or thirty times and eat them. Every time (you) eat, do not overfill. (You) should reduce (your intake) by 3-5 mouthfuls and still (feel) wanting (food.) This is good. To be full at one meal only obstructs the passage of breath, it does not allow the passage to communicate and hinders the daily exercise. Avoid especially grease, fats, sticky or greasy food, raw vegetables, turnips, stale and stinking (food), etc. Do not eat meat or fish dishes at all.

In the first thirty or fifty days, one is able not to be hungry. If (one) is still thinking of food, one should harmonize the breath. The stomach is gradually thus nourished and moistened, and (one) does not think of the hundred flavors. What was said of eating porridge and dumplings can be taken at will. When you want to eat, just eat at your convenience. Do not rely on this schedule daily as to when and what to eat. In general this should be the order of eating. One should obtain natural firmness and follow convenience. Eat repeatedly one meal of flavorless boiled rice since it is good anyhow.

In the beginning of the ingesting of breath, the three cooking vessels should communicate and while the appetite increases, the five viscera should be in harmony (with each other); the sweet juice (the saliva) should thus be produced. This is the jade pool (of the Yellow Court Canon, it is in the mouth) and it should be beautiful; when eating, food would seem sweet and attractive to a sick person who is recovering and is greedy for food without knowing satiation, and thinks that all the food is delicious. One must be moderate. (Otherwise), if one indulges, one will encounter great harm. Examine and calculate well the food (you eat.)

Any food contains some kind of poison. The five flavors, too, have warm breath. Therefore, after every meal, you should open your mouth and do the Ho_1 exhalation till it is felt that the heat of the breath inside your mouth has abated. Then for a long time no sickness will bother (you.) Moreover, (you) must be sparing of salt, the acrid and the sour. Do not eat them. In the beginning it is difficult. For the (first) ten or twenty days, the saliva juice flows from the magic spring, and this is not possible if salty or acrid (foods) enter (the body.)

As you are ingesting the breath, the five viscera are moistened, the proper breath goes down and removes, to the utmost, the stale and evil breath. Once the stale and evil breath has leaked out below, salty and acrid food will injure your clean stomach. You should not eat the food that is (too) cold, or (too) hot, sticky, greasy, raw or hard. Even only indulging in eating one mouthful (of such), where it stays, it will make you perceive a slight pain. After you have achieved the deep merit, you will naturally know this. Eat only things that are (well) cooked and soft. They are excellent. As (said) before, when the meal is over, immediately breathe out with the Ho_1 exhalation.

Each time you eat, take twenty or thirty grains of raw pepper with water. Then eat. If, after eating you perceive painful fullness, it is good to eat again ten or twenty grains of pepper. The virtue of pepper is that it makes the three cooking vessels communicate, it chases down the evil air, and it helps to break down and remove the old food. When regulating the proper breath, if the breath inbetween the heart and the chest is observed as stuffy, then hold two or three grains of pepper in your mouth. The stuffiness is immediately dispersed. Such is the virtue of pepper that it cannot be recounted (enough.) If you suddenly feel full or stuffy, sit down quietly and harmonize (the breath.) The stuffiness will immediately leak downward.

The old book states, "Solidify the breath. Do not let it leak out below." Formerly, beginning practitioners solidified the breath according to this saying. In a short while, the stomach (feels) stuffy so that one feels anxiously close to death. There are two holes below communicating above with the mouth and the nose, so that there are entrances and exits above and below in contact with each other. If the five viscera have stale and evil breath, it must exit below. (So) what is there to solidify? If it is solidified, breath does not flow and exit.

If breath does not flow and exit, then pain is felt. If, therefore, the stale breath does not exit and the fresh breath enters, the two breaths are mutually clashing with each other and this will do harm. Do not solidify (the breath.) It is better to have it flow and exit.

Each day, drink also one or two small cups of wine on an empty stomach according to your natural disposition. That is greatly wonderful. Try not to get nauseated. If you are able to drink daily three to five small cups (of wine), it will greatly assist the breath way (TAO.) Still, the wine must be pure and good so that you can bear drinking it. Don't take much. As soon as vomiting happens, the breath will not be even for days. If, on the occasion of a happy meeting, you want to drink much, there is a method (to do it.) The reason why men drink wine and get stupidly drunk, depressed and confused, is that wine contains the poison of fermenting yeast. As soon as poisonous air enters the four limbs, men get drunk. To drink correctly, (do as follows): When five or ten people sit at a table, passing often the cup to you, open your mouth and exhale with the Ho_1 (breath) seven or eight breaths after having drunk one cup. Then the wine poison exits and is dissipated. When wine cups arrive at the same time, then open your mouth greatly and exhale with Ho_1. If you take a cup at a time at will, just exhale subtly. In general, if you breathe rapidly, connect it with exhaling the Ho_1 to escort the breath out. If you are able to harmonize and manage (breath) unceasingly during the entire feast, then it is said that, for one who can (normally) drink three liters in a (feast) day, doing like this you might be able to drink ten liters and still be sober and free from inebriation, and, at the same time still not lose the wine taste. Though you would be drinking the whole day long, (the taste) would not diminish.

One can wait till after one wakes up to do the rinsing and swallowing (of saliva) and the regulating and managing (of the breath) as before. One still feels as usual. If suddenly there is air to exit below unexpectedly, maybe during a normal meal or when seated across from a guest, maybe when riding a horse, or when facing an honored relative; when the air comes, how could this be handled? One must let it leak out below according to convenience. If the air is shut up and does not leak out, then it goes in the wrong direction to the upper viscera. It will be stirringly painful in the stomach. If the heart and the rib (cage) are disturbed, such (a pain) would then not be dissipated for a long time.

One should give vent to the disordered breath and the stuffy pain inside. If one is too busy, due to the public or private affairs, to nourish one's life, then one should not eat meat or fish or (any of) the strong smelling vegetables. Then even if one lets the air leak out below, the air still does not have a very stinking smell. And, if one has cut off cereals there is still no stinking smell, even if one or two leaks come out.

Also, when there is unclean, bad air, or any serious illness, it is not to be confronted. It injures deeply the correct breath. If one must suddenly pass through a market place and encounter smelly air, one should then block the breath when passing through. Otherwise, one should drink (some) wine so as to have the wine breath and eat a little bit of pungent food, in order to be able to ward off the bad smell. If the bad breath has entered and one perceives (oneself) unquiet and insecure, then one must harmonize the breath to get rid (of the smell.)

Also, don't cry out loud, weep or wail. When you may not avoid the human affairs, which require mourning, cry a little and do not sob too much.

If breath rushes up unexpectedly against the throat (eructations, N.T.), do not indulge it to go upward. Swallow it down, then breathe in again to get breath and swallow it. It will settle within fifteen swallowings. As before, use your hands to massage it down to disperse it.

Keep (some) pepper inside the mouth and drink wine to dissipate such. If there is suddenly some difficulty in swallowing (the breath), do not force the swallowing, it will cause the upper cooking vessel to be obstructed. You should will for the breath to disperse and you should examine yourself presently. If breath does not disperse properly, do not eat. After having carelessly overeaten, do not swallow (the breath.) If you swallow the breath, it will be obstructed by the food and will not be able to go down. That will cause sickness. Cease any breathing through the mouth or nose at each swallowing. After the panting is settled, use the mind to escort it outward. Observe the breath. On the left side it passes twenty-four ridges. As it passes, you can hear them. (It is) like water dripping down a hole. The sound is most clear and rhythmic. If it does not make the sound, it is because you ate something greasy or have not followed the proper sequence (of practice.) If breath does not disperse soon, and if you still ingest breath, it will press (the old breath.) It perforce produces sickness. You must be especially careful.

All the beginners in the ingesting (of the breath method) desire its virtue greedily. They all impose upon their breath and think that the more they practice ingesting the better. They add maybe ten or twenty breaths every day. As long as they perceive that they are temporarily safe and steady, they add furthermore thirty or fifty breath swallowings. They think that advancing gradually on a daily basis is a gain. They do not know that breath has not yet been communicating and moistening. Hence illness is caused. There is sickness in the abdomen, yet one does not know it until the symptoms of disquietude show. One augments the number of ingesting daily, and the accumulation becomes coagulating. Once it achieves coagulating, breath is painful on both flanks. There is difficulty in eventually prescribing proper medicine.

If, however, the accomplishment is attained gradually in the long time of three years, even if there is some offense, it cannot hinder the ingesting of the breath. Even if one has achieved more than one thousand swallowings daily, one is not afraid. If the ninth year is reached, the merit finally does not diminish anymore and the joints connect mutually.

The Yellow Court Canon states, "Thousands and hundreds will naturally connect together. Ones and tens will be arranged like rows of mountain ranges." It is talking about the flesh and the bones mutually connecting together. If the five viscera are (nourished) like this, one can afterwards enter water and not be drowned. (One's) inside breath does not exit and the outside air does not enter. Keep in this state for ten or twenty days. Then one will have no fear at all of great cold or great heat. Regardless of being old or young, the cold or the heat will not last long.

Generally, in ingesting breath, one should tighten the fists. However, a beginner, whose breath has not circulated yet, should not tighten the fists. Wait till half a year or one hundred days later when one perceives that one's breath flows freely and one's palms sweat, then one may tighten the fists.

The Yellow Court Canon states, "If the three passes are shut and blocked, stop tightening the fists. Hold in the mouth and rinse the golden fountain of sweet water. Swallow the jade flower. By following this (procedure), one achieves not to be hungry and the Three Worms die. The will is constantly at ease and this brings delight and prosperity".

The sea of breath is below the navel. Because in everybody the three cooking vessels do not communicate, the (ordinary) panting (type of) breathing does not pass beyond the navel. Another reason why the panting breath does not settle is that the breath does not go down but presses only in the upper cooking vessel, the heart or the chest. At the start, a beginner's upper cooking vessel does not communicate in the first five or ten days. From the tenth to the twentieth day, one will perceive the breath passing through the holes in the joints and entering the sea of breath. The sound "yu-yu" is heard.

It is thus subtly perceived (how) breath is circulating. The breath reaches the sea of breath and it is lengthened since the breath condition is harmonious and good. The old book is also not detailed (enough.) It makes only a (passing) mention about relaxing the prohibitions. Veteran practitioners mostly follow that and hence injure the correct breath. The middle way (TAO) is empty. Do not let (though) this be the only guiding principle. It is because I had experienced what was harmful or beneficial that I repeated (here) the details.

When harmonizing the breath, the breathing must be done carefully, so that it is fine and inaudible. If it is audible, it is coarse and harmful to the correct breath. (Exhale with) Ho_1, only when the heat is great. Don't be afraid of a little (heat.) If it is perceived that the heat has settled, then you should regulate it carefully and finely. It is only proper for a beginning practitioners, who still does not understand the swallowing, to swallow just one breath. At each swallowing, bulge your mouth like a great drum to lead the (inside inhaled, N.T.) breath to fill the mouth. Then swallow it when it is imminent (to exit.) The upper cooking vessel will communicate after you understand the swallowing. Then you do not need to bulge your mouth. Only shut breath off and close your mouth with determination. Don't breathe yet. To swallow in succession, do three swallowings before one exhalation, then swallow again. Attend thus to swallow to reach eight, nine swallowings per exhalation. You may reach twenty swallowings per exhalation or thirty swallowings (before) exhaling once.

This means that the breath goes down into the sea of breath and eases up the tendons and the vessels in order to communicate. At this stage, you are to be careful about the proper condition of the breath and you should examine whether the breath cycle is long or short, circulating or not. Also (in the beginning), don't seek to prolong and to do much swallowing in this way. Much swallowing is not good (either) since it is not peaceful and firm. To obtain peacefulness and firmness, for each shutting of the mouth, undertake (only) one swallowing. When the swallowed breath enters, use the mind to escort (it) down to reach the sea of breath. Then do further swallowing without exhaling. Practice this constantly. The beginner in the swallowing of (the breath) does not know either how to regulate the conditions of the breath. He has to use the mind to escort (the breath down.) It is (only) later that you know how to escort the breath gradually. Cut off (any other) thought, be without thought and indulge in swallowing at will; the breath will take its own position. Then you don't have to use your hands to massage and the mind to escort (the breath.)

The Book (TAO TE CHING, Chapter II, N.T.) states, "What is the wordless teaching? The Ten Thousand Things work without action (WU WEI.) Living without action, they still achieve the merit. Yet when the merit is achieved, they do not claim any credit." The mind of the one who teaches without words is in accordance with nature. He has no calculated action nor thoughts.

The reason why the five viscera and the six receptacles nourish life, yet do not possess, is that they produce the breath of the TAO in the body, which does not in turn presume upon their existence. The merit is achieved with certainty, yet it is not claimed. The practice cannot be observed from the outside. If it could be looked at, it would be known by others. If it were known by others, then the self produces. If the self produces then fame could be achieved. If fame is achieved, than calamity would come. If calamity comes, then breath dies. If breath dies, then that is destruction.

The Yellow Court Canon states, therefore, "If you are able to understand the One, ten thousand affairs will be concluded, naturally."

The reason why I talked about the order of eating and the timing of ingesting breath at midnight, the fifth watch, and the three periods daily, is to record it all for the beginners who have not yet understood it. After one understands it thoroughly, one can handle matters carefully and approach them at one's convenience. However, one should not adhere to it obstinately. Obstinate adherence produces anxiety. If anxiety is produced then the mind is tied. If the mind is tied, then it toils. If the mind is over-burdened, the virtue declines. Bear it in mind! Bear it in mind!

The "Hsien Ching" (The Immortality Book) states, "When man approaches his end, he begins to love his body. (Only) after the crime has been committed, he thinks about converting himself to be a good person. (Only) after sickness has come, he strives towards obtaining the remedy for it."

Once the heavenly net (of retribution) has been (widely) cast, there is no use to regret. The virtuous men and the superior scholars, therefore, treasure the life that is not endangered yet. They dread what is not yet a calamity and they heal what is not yet a sickness. These are the genuine and superior scholars. That is what genuine protection and love is (all) about.

It says, moreover, "(There is) youth, middle age and old age. Youth is from over twenty (years old) to (somewhere) under thirty (years old.) Middle age is from over the age of forty to (somewhere) under fifty. Old age is (when) one is in his sixties and seventies. Beyond eighty the harm is set in and settled.

"If when young, man is humble and becomes aware and cognizant of the principle (TAO), he recognizes and penetrates the profound and the subtle. His body is solid, (his) bones are strong. His muscles are perfect. His flesh manifests fullness. If he starts his mind in the way (TAO), he will for sure achieve the virtue.

"The middle-aged become aware of the way (TAO) somewhat late. Their muscles, flesh, bones, and marrow are all at half (strength.) (Being) in between advancing and retreating, the (overall) effect (of the practice) is (relatively) slight.

"In the aged, who are in their sixties and seventies, their bone marrow, their muscles and blood vessels are at twenty or thirty percent (strength.) The virtue is at sunset. They might still be able to be saved. Beyond the eighties, the brain is exhausted, the (bone) marrow is used up, the ten thousand passes are dry and rotted out, the soul is fading away, and the breath is dying. They are a walking corpse, a ghost on foot, incapable of being rescued.

"The ancient worthies and superior scholars knew, therefore, that it is difficult to nourish the mind and the heart during the "candle-in-the-wind" (old age) years. therefore, they put away vulgar toiling and love the body as the (foremost) treasure. Consequently, (they) idle (their) ambitions and retire to remote caves to pacify the mind and return to the way (TAO.) The way (TAO) is the breath. This breath is the root of the body."

Fish separated from water die. If man has lost the way (TAO), then it is difficult to (become) perfect. To devote attention to nourishing life is (but) nourishing breath. To nourish breath is (but) paying attention to guard the essence (or the sperm.) If the essence and the breath are both intact, they are called the genuine jewels. Furthermore, men have three elixir fields (TAN-T'IEN) (called): the Upper Original, the Middle Original and the Lower Original. The Upper Original elixir field is the NI-WAN (MUD PILL) which is the brain. One (of its) names is TI HSIANG, (the supreme god country, i.e., heaven), The Middle Original is the central TAN-T'IEN (elixir field) which is the heart. It is also called CHIANG KUNG-CHEN-JEN, (the scarlet palace of the genuine man.) The Lower Original is the lower elixir field (TAN-T'IEN) which is the sea of breath, also called CHING-MEN (the door of the essence.) These three originals have one spirit each. If any of the spirits is deficient, then breath is deficient and the essence leaks.

If leaves fall off, and a tree rots, it loses its luster. Therefore, the former worthies who aspired to the Tao (Way) all treasured the breath and guarded the essence in order to perfect themselves.

Refining the Breath

The method to refine the breath is as follows: Take advantage of the free time to ingest the breath, go to a quiet, unoccupied room. Undo your hair, undress and cover yourself with a quilt. Lie down with your face looking straight up, your feet and hands must be spread apart, don't tighten the fists. The sides of the clean mat should hang down to the floor. Straighten and comb your hair so it is loose and natural and let it fall on the mat. Then harmonize the breath. If the breath condition is proper and if you feel stuffy, then open your mouth and exhale. At the first exhalation, if you pant hurriedly, then harmonize the breath seven, eight or ten times. Then the breath comes and the panting breath will be settled. When settled, refine it even more. In this way, if you have time, refine it properly ten times and then stop. In the beginning, you should be aware that the breath has not circulated yet. It is still clogged under the skin. That is not good. If you have more time, you should refine the (breath) some more by increasing the refinements by five or six. Progress gradually in adding refinements. There is no limit. What is the principle (of this?) When one has ingested breath for a short time and the effect is gradually achieved, the joints will be communicating and the hair pores open up. If twenty or thirty refinements are reached, the body is then moistened throughout and perspiration appears.

When this sign is obtained, it is the verification of the achieved effect. The beginner in refining should stop once breath does communicate and the moistening (perspiration, N.T.) is achieved. It is good if one progresses gradually in perspiring.

Lie down quietly and serenely. Don't rise up soon to rush into the wind. Should a sick person perspire (like this), he should rest well and long, obtain clean clothes to wear and retire in a place with no draft. Walk slowly! Talk little! Love breath! Be thrifty with affairs! Think clearly! The body will, consequently, be light and the hundreds of arteries will flow and irrigate. The four limbs communicate pleasantly. The Yellow Court Canon therefore states, "The thousand calamities disappear and the hundred illnesses are healed. One does not fear being injured by the ferocious tiger or the wolf. In addition, one gets rid of old age and extends life forever."

The practitioners refine the breath daily, starting at night and noon, whenever there is a convenient time when the soul's natural disposition is clear and pleasant. Then follow the previous order by sitting erect to nourish and swallow. Work diligently. Do not become lazy, this may lead to sleepiness. If you become sleepy or feel stuffy, you should sleep rather than insist on sitting. If you insist on sitting, then you confuse your will. If the will is bewildered, then breath is disordered and it loses the correct way (TAO.) The beginner in the ingesting (of the breath) does not have the correct breath yet, (he) is consequently confused and sleepy.

After a period of time, you will no more be so much confused. When refining breath, don't do it daily. Practice it every five or ten days, when you have excessive leisure, and when you perceive that there is no pleasant communication and that your entire body is troubled and (feels) stuffy. Daily practice may bring no effect. Don't do it often.

The Method of Abandoning Breathing

The nourishment of breath (means to be able to) abandon breathing. You should wait for the whole body to be quiet and harmonious, and the mind to be without ambition or thought. Either sitting or lying down, harmonize the breath by breathing through the proper "door" and "window". Staying still, abandon your body like abandoning a (piece of clothing, N.T.) on a bed. You will feel as if you are without muscles, without bones, without a soul, and without perception. Relax the mind and relax the ears. Just like abandoned clothes the ruler is suddenly in deep silence. Being in deep silence, you liberate the form, abandon the body, cleanse the soul and refine the breath. Then the hundred joints open up and stretch. The joints and the arteries communicate pleasantly, the saliva juice flows and pours down. In this state, swallow down ten breaths or twenty breaths.

In swallowing (and refining), one should, moreover, definitely be able to breathe at ease so that there is no mutual wrangling with the will. After a long time, the breath exits through hundreds of hair pores rather than having to use again the exhalation through the mouth. Stop even if an eighty or ninety percent (result) is obtained. Then harmonize (the breath) again for several tens of breaths up to more than one hundred breaths. If you suddenly breathe rapidly, you should hold a little breath in your mouth and swallow it. Then harmonize the breath. In harmonizing, you will feel as if the four limbs, the skin, the flesh, the joints are being bathed.

Whenever you have leisure time, do not lie face up; lie, rather, on the side. Lying or sitting or standing, you are to practice to abandon the breath and the body. Its effect will advance daily. The essence will be filled and the breath will be perfected. The upper soul will quiet down and the lower soul will settle. Thought will be at leisure and the aspirations will be quite profound. The way (TAO) will be prosperous and the attributes peaceful. The Three Corpses will automatically pass away, and the six defilements will also be destroyed

The Yellow Court Canon, therefore, states, "Being at leisure and without (any) involvement in affairs, the body will be quiet. To abide in nothingness relies totally upon leisure."

If you can nourish only the breath in doing nothing (WU WEI), abandon the body and the mind and let go of the form and the thoughts, so you may be united with the way (TAO.) Then you will know (its) different manifestations naturally.

The Yellow Court Canon says: "Highly respecting non-action (WU WEI), the upper (HUN) and the lower (P'O) souls are quiet. (Enjoying) a pure and quiet vision, the souls talk to me". The meaning is what (was talked about) above. In practicing the abandonment of the breath, if you suddenly feel that the entire body is not harmonious or the body is blocked, and the conditions of the breath are not harmonious, then do the abandoning of the breath. Regardless of whether lying down or sitting, cleanse the soul and abandon the breath. Appease the thought to be silent and calm the mind for long. Then stay still and perceive how breath flows everywhere. There should be no place where there is deficiency.

The method to block the breath

The man possessing superior wisdom has a determined will power and high aspiration. When he nourishes and manages by himself, the merit of the effect bestowed is not insignificant. His soul is settled and the breath is harmonized. He has interrupted (the source) of outside illness. For a man of average wisdom, maybe because he has still not concluded his personal affairs, maybe because his mind is caught in-between advancing or withdrawing, he does not abide by the prohibitions (necessary) to harmonize and nourish (the breath.) He acts against the rules, and his breath is blocked and inharmonious. (Instead of having good results from nourishing), he, on the contrary causes disasters. If thus he has physical hardship, he is to enter a quiet room, lie down face up, harmonize the breath to the proper condition, spread out his hands and feet which should be away from (the body) four or five inches. As usual, the mat on which (he) lies down should be thick and soft. During the winter months, the quilt should be warm. He should quiet his mind and be peaceful. He is then to swallow breath and block the breath immediately. He should not move his mouth and his nose. He should use the mind to think of where the ailment is, and use the will to pour (the breath) onto it. If the breath (which is held) is to the extreme, then exhale. After finishing the exhaling, block the breath again.

For each blocking, at the first exhalation, if the breath is rapid, harmonize it six, seven times. When breath is harmonized and agreeable, block it some more and think constantly of working at the trouble spot maybe ten, maybe twenty, thirty, forty, or fifty (times.) Stop if perspiration is observed and circulation is opened up and flowing and irrigating properly. If you still do not feel well, do it daily in the fifth night watch (3 - 5 AM) or at night. You should work on the ailment often, till a difference is observed.

If the pain is in your left hand, have the mind enter straight to your left hand. If it is in your right hand, enter straight into your right hand. If in your head, let the mind go straight up to your head. You should observe the efficacy (of this) obviously. Then you will know that the mind is able to employ the breath. The breath follows the will which commands the breath like magic. There should not be grief, sorrow or joy. For if the mind is grieving, then it injures the soul, while if euphoric, it loses (the train) of thought. If you have an illness, you should do as described above. Then you will remove such (pain) for sure.

The method by which to abstain from (eating) cereals

He who wants to abstain from (eating) cereals should rely at first only on the nourishing practice as described above. After three years, the five viscera will be nourished, the body will be firm, the flesh will be full, hundreds of spirits return back to their respective positions, the blood circulates, and the breath way (TAO) is wide and pleasant and flows throughout, without any obstruction. You are able to become light and feel renewed daily. If you advance gradually like this you will have no use for the breath of the five flavors, you will not think of food constantly. If you have to interrupt such, there is no difficulty in doing so.

The worldly man is avaricious of pleasure and profits. He is unable to interrupt thoughts. He is therefore searching for many (different) prescriptions in books about drugs that could be taken in order to interrupt (the eating) of cereals. At first when the drugs enter the stomach, it seems they temporarily fill it up. But when the effect of the medicine disappears, hunger appears. This is a vicious circle. Moreover, if the mind is constantly hooked on the medicine, longing for harmony in the ceaseless daily affairs, the person's strength will be weakened and his wisdom will be exhausted. There will be increasing annoyance and grief. Even if medicine is taken, how could one suddenly cut off the cereals without inviting disasters? Maybe eating fruits can assist one's strength, or taking medicine can satiate one's appetite. One should try to harmonize (breath) more and regulate (it) so as to nourish breath and pacify thoughts. The toil and labor of seeking medicine and the distress of brewing it diligently month after month wastes a person's energy. How can he reverse old age, and restore his age?

How could it be called abstinence, if people only abstain from rice? Among them, there are the inferior scholars, who are unable to cut off the worldly affairs suddenly. If they take medicine to help (the practice), it is (indeed) of little benefit. A superior man would not proceed in this way (TAO.) In general, for ingesting breath, once the virtue is achieved, one must abstain from cereals. Whenever the stomach is empty, one should swallow breath. Regardless of morning or night, there is no hindrance or obstruction. If one has to swallow, just swallow. There is no limit of number either. If the practitioner himself observes that the conditions require him to stop, then he must not do a lot of swallowing. The practitioner himself should understand when he can ingest for long (that he has) to be able to cut off (eating) cereals. I will not bother to write it all down. If, in the beginning of the practice, one wishes to take medicine to help along the ingestion of breath, it will also do. However, most of the medicine-takers end up not ingesting breath, but with the medicine becoming the main thing. HUANG T'ING CHING (The Yellow Court Canon) says, "The substances of the hundreds of grains are the hobgoblins of the earth. The five flavors, externally beautiful, are (but) foul smelling evil demons. They stink and disturb the soul and reduce the Embryonic Breath to naught. How can one reverse old age and return to infancy?"

There are still government officials who abide in splendor and prosperity, and whose worldly affairs have not yet been ended. Even if they long for the way (TAO) and meditate on the genuine, they cannot cut out the (worldly) aspiration. If they still confine their mind on years and months, it is in vain for them to accumulate their diligence. If they just wait for the time to come to cut off their lust, they are wasting time while declining into the sunset years (of their lives.) How should one then be able to have a solid accomplishment, without gradually progressing in nourishing (the breath)?

The man who holds a government office is compelled to pay attention to official business and he is unable to rely daily on the three periods for the nourishing (practice.) He should then rinse his mouth and swallow the saliva juice according to the previous method, at midnight or in the fifth watch when waking up from sleep. He should harmonize the breath and obtain the proper breath conditions. In order to rid the lower cooking vessel of its heat, he should then try to swallow forty or fifty swallowings. (For his general practice) he should start with 10 or 20 swallowings, then he is to add 5 swallowings daily till he reaches 50 swallowings. Then in the daytime, even if he has to attend to the official affairs, he can preserve the genuine and establish (his) will power. Even this little will do!

The end of the T'AI CH'ING T'IAO CH'I CHING.

CHEN CH'I HUAN YÜAN MING THE CARVED (TEXT) ON THE RECOVERY OF THE GENUINE BREATH, WITH A COMMENTARY BY CH'IANG MING TZU

(Tao Tsang Vol. VII, p.802; Harvard Yenching 131; Wieger 261)

ONE BREATH, UNDIVIDED.

"One" is the spontaneity of TAO. "Breath" is what the One produces, (while) "UNDIVIDED" is the HUN-TUN (the primordial chaos) which is undivided. Here what is meant is that though the "ONE BREATH" follows the Great TAO to become designated (named), it is the breath of the primordial chaos, which has not yet made a distinction between the pure and the turbid. This then is the nameless producing a name, and which (in its turn) produces the ten thousand things. The TAO book (TAO TE CHING) says, "The nameless is the origin of heaven and earth, while the named is the mother (a cause) to the ten thousand things". The nameless means the TAO. The named means the breath. What is called the TAO is the father (ancestor) of the ONE BREATH, while what is called ONE BREATH is the mother (cause) of the ten thousand things. What has image and form can not be produced without being caused by the ONE BREATH.

Therefore, nourishing life is to value TAO. Practicing the TAO is to emphasize breath. It means that breath is the root of the essence and of the soul, the life source and the ruler of the spirit. If a man knows the method to nourish the breath, he is able to become an immortal. Therefore, the Yellow Court Canon says, "Coming out from the clear and going into the obscure, the two breaths are brilliant. If you can encounter them, you will ascend to heaven." It also says, "Why not ingest the breath which is the extremely harmonious essence, and thus, not entering death, abide in the Yellow Repose?" Its meaning from above is clear.

THREE FORCES OF IDENTICAL ORIGIN.

Heaven, earth and man are the three forces. "Of identical origin" means that the three forces all abide in the same origin of the primordial chaos (HUN-TUN.)

(THOUGH) THE CLEAR AND THE TURBID ARE ALREADY DIFFERENT,

"The clear" is heaven, "the turbid" is the earth, "already" means in the end, "different" means distinct. The meaning is that the breath of the primordial chaos (HUN-TUN) gets divided and discriminated. The clear breath rises, therefore, and becomes heaven, while the turbid breath sinks down to be the earth, and man is inbetween. Hence a difference.

THEY ALL KEEP THE ORIGINAL AND THE ESSENCE RESPECTIVELY.

"The Original" is the Original Breath, "the essence" is the essence of the Original Breath. It says that heaven, earth and man all nurture their respective essence of the Original Breath.

THE LAWS OF HEAVEN RESEMBLE MINE,

This means that for the one who is nurturing the original and the essence, the laws and the image of heaven are still the same as those of man.

WHILE MY LAWS RESEMBLE THOSE OF HEAVEN.

This means that man's laws resemble heaven's laws in order to achieve a perfect form. One may ask, "Since the laws of heaven resemble mine, and my laws resemble heaven's laws, as previously said, the heavenly TAO (principle) should never undermine the human TAO. Why then is there Life and Death?"

I reply, "Though the heavenly TAO (principle) is the fundamental pivot of the whole mechanism, it is pure, void, and intentionless. If pure, void and intentionless, the Original Breath circulates naturally. If the Original Breath circulates naturally, the five elements are unhindered. If the five elements are unhindered, there is no punishment or destruction. If there is no punishment or destruction, this is the great emptiness. If this is the great emptiness, then all is contained in the TAO and identical to it. This is what is meant by not undermining".

I further reply, "The fact that man undergoes living and dying is not different from the heavenly TAO. It is only caused by man himself. What I mean by 'caused by man himself' is explained as follows: From the time of his parents' intercourse during which the essence and the breath coagulate, and give rise to a body that is born, man experiences sadness, tears, happiness, anger, grief, and joy. Gradually, his mouth is greedy for the five tastes, his ears delight with the five tones, his eyes gaze on the five colors, and his mind is involved in the five desires. No change takes place without these. Above are the four things which all caused his mind to change and move. Once there is mind, there is no purity and voidness. When there is no purity and voidness, man loses the TAO. If man loses the TAO, the same (happens) to the ten thousand species. All things are alike in that they give themselves wantonly to life and death, and they let themselves be destined to rot and decay. Some are like a sparkling fire, some resemble bubbles. When they exist, they exist temporarily; when they disappear, they disappear right away. This is caused by man and not by the great TAO. If man could be of a mind-less mind, of an eye-less eye, of a taste-less taste, of a view-less view, of a passion-less passion, of an understanding void of understanding, and of a change-less change, he would then be in harmony with the light and would blend with the dust. Being pure and constant, he would be identical to the TAO. Why, then could he not extend his life to be "as long as heaven?"

MY DESTINY IS WITHIN MYSELF.

This means that man's fate of living and dying is caused by man himself. If man (only) was able to know the way (TAO) of naturalness, to change and move the breath of the original harmony, to swallow the two external bright views (THE SUN AND THE MOON, N. T.), and to ingest the five internal (grain) germs (the breath of the five viscera, N.T,) then, when in action, he could regulate the hundred spirits, and, when in quietude, he could calm down the five viscera. Hence cold, heat, hunger and thirst would be unable to encroach upon him, and the five weapons and the white sword (the five tastes N. T.) could not approach. Death and life would be in his hands and the transformations would be caused by his mind. The earth would be unable to bury him and heaven would be unable to kill him. This is what is meant by "my destiny is within myself."

AND (IT IS) NOT OF HEAVEN.

This means that man's destiny of living and dying is not caused by heaven.

BY ABUSING IT, ONE IS ABOUT TO DIE YOUNG,

This means that the person who abuses the Original Breath will have the adverse result of dying young. He should, therefore, follow a bright teacher who will teach him so he can apply (this teaching); otherwise he is about to reach death at a tender age.

WHILE PERFECTING IT, IT LENGTHENS LIFE.

This means that if a person understands the principles of the Original Breath, he prolongs and lengthens his life.

(WHEN) BREATH IS HARMONIOUS, THEN THE BODY IS STILL.

"Breath" is the Original Breath. "The body" means the body frame. This means that if the Original Breath is pliant and harmonious, the body form is naturally quiet; if the body form is still, the breath is naturally harmonious.

(WHILE) HOLDING THE ONE, THE SOUL IS RELAXED.

"The One" is the one Embryonic Breath. "The soul" is the spiritual form. What is meant here is that if a man is able to hold only the one breath, his spiritual form will be naturally at ease. The soul is the son of the breath, and (the breath) is (therefore) the mother of the soul. If a person knows how to respect the mother, then the son is not far. Knowing how to nurture the parent, his soul is undispersed. His soul is not being scattered away, it is in natural agreement with TAO (the Way.) It is a natural (phenomenon) like water flowing downward or fire flames (shooting) upward, or clouds obeying the dragon and winds obeying the tiger, etc.

THE EFFICACIOUS MUSHROOM IS IN THE BODY,

"The efficacious mushroom" is the fungus (of immortality.) "In the body" means inside the human body. This points to the Original Breath.

(AND) NOT ON A FAMOUS MOUNTAIN.

What has to be gathered is not to be found on a famous mountain.

RETURN TO THE ONE (BY) UPHOLDING HARMONY,

"The One" is the one soul. "Harmony" is the harmonious breath. In the previous section it was, "While holding the One, the soul is relaxed." Here it says to return to the one soul and guard the harmonious breath. This means that if the soul and the breath nurture each other mutually, they are thought as a joint continuum which is uninterrupted and without end.

THE PRINCIPLE ACCORDS WITH THE DOUBLE MYSTERY.

"The Principle" is the TAO principle. "The Double Mystery" is the further mystery. This means that if man is able to know how to return to the one soul, and yet nurture the harmonious breath, this is called "'The mystery of the mystery." (From the First Chapter of the TAO TE CHING, N.T.)

ESSENCE TAKEN TO ITS OUTER LIMITS IS SPIRIT,

"The essence" is the essential breath. "The spirit" is the soul's brightness. This means that if man obtains the method of embracing the Original and of holding the ONE, then the essential breath is fully filled up, and he can be in communication with the spiritual world.

AND THE EPITOME OF THE SOUL IS DIVINITY.

"The soul" is the ONE soul. "The Divinity" is man's divine communication. Here this means that if man successfully arrives at the way (TAO) of embracing the

Original and holding the ONE, the thirty six thousand souls will never leave him and he will then naturally be in communication with the divine. (The thirty six thousand souls probably refer to a prolonged life span of at least 100 years of 360 days each, or 36,000 days; thus a soul or spirit for each day, N.T.)

THE BREATH (TAKEN) TO ITS OUTER LIMITS IS PURITY, THE PURE BREATH IS THE SOUL, WHILE THE TURBID BREATH IS THE FORM (OR BODY.)

The "breath" is the Original Breath, "purity" is the purity of the void. Here is meant that if the Original Breath is (present) in the extreme, the turbid breath is naturally dismissed (or scattered) and man will be pure and simple.

THE CAUSE OF DECLINE IS BREATH,

This means that man's bodily decline is always due to the decline of the breath.

AND THE CAUSE OF PROSPERITY IS BREATH (AS WELL.)

If man's breath is prosperous, then the body prospers.

THE CAUSE OF DESTRUCTION IS BREATH,

When man's breath is exhausted, then the body is destroyed.

AND THE CAUSE OF BIRTH IS ALSO BREATH.

The reason why man's body was born is always due to the union of the Original Breaths of vitality.

JOYS OR RAGES DISTURB THE BREATH,

This means that man's joys or angers all disturb the correct breath.

FEELINGS AND MOODS ENGAGE IN CONTENTIONS.

This means that as a consequence of man having joys and angers, the feelings and natural dispositions will engage in wranglings.

CONGESTION AND ISOLATION LEAD TO SICKNESS.

Previously it said that "Feelings and moods engage in contentions". That is the congestions and isolation of the Original Breath. If breath is congested and isolated, it leads to illness.

HOW COULD THE SOULS AND THE FORM BE PEACEFUL?

"The souls" are the ten thousand spirits. "The form" is the bodily form. "How could (they) be peaceful," means that the whole body cannot be at peace.

REFINE THE YANG AND MELT THE YIN,

"Refine" is like heating and smelting. "The YANG" is the Yang breath.

"Melt" is like fusing. "The Yin" is the Yin breath. It was said before that the soul and the body can not attain quietude and peace. Here it says to refine the Yang and to melt the Yin. It is the entrance to capturing and controlling. It is the method of harmonizing and managing.

In general, all those who seek immortality and learn the way (TAO) to nourish and nurture must know how to heat and refine the Yang breath, melt and fuse the Yin evil. They are then able to prolong life. Moreover human illnesses are caused in general by the five tastes which may grow and destroy the body. When beginning to ingest breath, the fire (for heating) is accumulated in the mind first so that it can heat the entire body. Once the heating is completed, one is to ingest the breath according to the method. No disease will resist being cured. Kuang Cheng Tzu said, "Accumulate the fire and use it to burn the five poisons," "The five poisons" are the five tastes. When the five poisons are exhausted, one is able to prolong life.

YOUR BREATH CIRCULATES NATURALLY, YOUR SOUL IS NATURALLY DIVINE.

This means that after the Yin breath is dissipated and exhausted, the Yang breath circulates naturally.

USE WHAT IS RIGHT TO SEND AWAY THE WRONG,

"The right" (or the correct) is the correct breath. "The wrong" is the evil breath. It says to use the correct breath to send away the evil breath.

AND YOUR MISFORTUNE WILL SUBSIDE NATURALLY,

"Subside" means there is no misfortune. It was said before to use the correct breath to send away the evil breath. It is like hot water being poured over snow, or using fire to melt away ice. Misfortune will naturally subside as before.

(SO THAT THE) CH'IEN AND K'UN ARE PURE AND CALM.

From now on, (the text) speaks about the order in the method of ingesting breath. "Ch'ien" stands for heaven. "K'un" stands for earth. This means that heaven and earth are as clear and pure as in a day without wind, clouds, fog, rain or snow.

AFTER THE TZU HOUR AND BEFORE THE WU HOUR,

"The Tzu hour" is at midnight, "The Wu hour" is noon. All training in inhalation and exhalation and in the ingestion of the Original Breath is usually entirely to be done between midnight and noon, when it is the time to train and ingest breath which is called the breath of the six periods of the Yang; (whereas) the time between noon and midnight when it is prohibited to train the breath and ingest the internal breath, is called the six periods of the Yin breath. Everything, consequently will be without any hindrance (if one is proceeding in such a manner, N.T.)

CLOSE YOUR EYES, SIT LEVEL,

Here (then) is the time when heaven is clear and pure: it is the time before the Wu hour, (11:00 A.M. - 1:00 P.M.) and after the TZU hour (11:00 P.M. to 1:00 A.M.) Here is the time to train breath and ingest (it.) Close your eyes, face south, and sit level, to harmonize and ingest the breath. This is the ordinary method.

TIGHTEN YOUR FISTS AND CLOSE YOUR EYES,

If you close your eyes and sit level, it is necessary to firmly tighten your fists and hold your thumbs. Close your eyes as if closing (them), and yet not completely closing them (the eyelids should be lowered, N.T.)

INHALE THROUGH THE THATCHED HUT,

"The thatched hut" is the nose. Inhale the outside air through the nose and very subtly conduct (it by swallowing it, N.T.) and fill "the sea of breath." If done over a long period of time, it is a wonder. This is called "inhaling the new".

AND EXHALE THROUGH THE HEAVEN'S GATE.

"Exhale" is expelling the breath. "The heaven's gate" is the mouth. Previously the inhaled outside breath had been led to enter "the sea of breath". After some time (the left-over air, N.T.) must be exhaled. This is designated as "exhaling the old".

THE BREATH SHOULD ENTER VERY SUBTLY.

"Very subtly" means that when the nose draws in the outside air, it should draw it very subtly so that the ear should not hear it. Being subtle and fine is the gate to life. Being rough is the road to death. The inhalation should, therefore, be done in a subtle and fine way (TAO.)

BREATHE OUT CONTINUOUSLY. USE THE THOUGHT TO LEAD THE BREATH.

This explains how the nose draws in the external air. One must use the thought to lead the external air properly to the sea of breath.

IT REVOLVES IN THE VISCERA AND THE RECEPTACLES.

This means that if one uses the will to guide the outside breath into "the sea of breath" and fill it, the breath in the five viscera and the six receptacles circulates naturally and goes slightly around, making a soft "ku, ku" sound.

EXHALE IT THEN WITH HO_1.

The "Ho_1" is the mouth making the Ho_1 (sound) when exhaling (the breath.) It was said above that air (should) revolve in the viscera and the receptacles. When air is (held) to the extreme, it must be exhaled with the Ho (sound.) One should not forcefully keep the air in.

LET THE BLOOD AND THE BREATH CIRCULATE THOROUGHLY.

This means that when the principle of breathing is practiced, the blood and the breath will be without congestion and obstruction.

IF IT IS NOT HARMONIOUS,

If it is untimely, the five viscera and the six receptacles are not harmonious.

SEND IT AWAY TO THE HEEL.

"Send it away" as is written above means that the correct sends away the evil. As for the heel, the NAN HUA CHING (The Southern Flower Book) says, "The breathing of all humans is (done) through the throat, while the breathing of the genuine man is (done) through the heel." The heel is the base of the foot. Moreover, the T'AI HSI CHING (Embryonic Breath Book) says, "The ordinary people's breathing is different from the genuine man's breathing. The ordinary man's breathing exits and enters through the throat. The genuine man's breathing (is taking place) inside the sea of breath. This is the root of the breath."

According to my understanding of WAI-CH'U, it is said that the "CHUNG-TZU" (rear of the foot) is called "CHUNG" (heel.) The heel is the base of the foot. What is meant here is that the heel is the root of the breath. The meaning of base is root. It means (that) "the sea of breath" is where man's life root is based. Therefore if (the breath) is not harmonious, in order to chase away the evil breath, do the Embryonic Breath (breathing) according to the method previously stated.

DO THE HO_1 EXHALATION FIVE OR SIX TIMES.

The "Ho$_1$" is one of the six breathing. This means that, in general, the breaths of the five viscera and the six receptacles are all connected to the heart. The heart is the host of the Ho$_1$ breath. To use the Ho$_1$ breathing is, therefore, the superior method. Once the Ho$_1$ breathing is concluded, ingest the breath and circulate it according to the proper method.

NONE OF THE DISEASES WILL NOT BE ALLEVIATED.

This means that when one does the Ho$_1$ breathing, no diseases will not be alleviated.

IF YOU DESIRE THE EMBRYONIC BREATH,

The coagulation of the breath (CH'I) is called the embryo. The exhaling and inhaling is called the breath. If the embryo coagulates inside the breath, the breath is then breathed inside the embryo and (the whole process) is called Embryonic Breath.

THE BREATHING EXERCISES (TAO YIN) COME FIRST.

Do this between the TZU (11:00 P.M. - 1:00 A M.) and the WU hours (11:00 A M. - 1:00 P.M.) Do it (as explained) before sitting level, holding your fists firmly closed and slightly closing your eyes.

YOUR ARTERIES AND VEINS ARE NOT CLOGGED,

This means that if one exercises with breathing first, the breath will not be blocked or stagnant in one's veins and arteries.

AND YOUR JOINTS WILL NOT BE TROUBLESOME.

This means that the breathing exercises with their vibrations and pull move the joints so the Original Breath will flow without any obstruction. This is why it says, "the joints will not be troublesome".

(ONE MAY MOVE) PERHAPS AS IF AIMING TO SHOOT DOWN AN EAGLE,

From here on down the method of the Taoist exercises is (described) about how to lead and guide (the breath.) It is said here to turn the body in the gesture of aiming at shooting down an eagle.

AND TWIST THE SIDES OF YOUR BODY AND BEND (YOUR ARMS TO FORM, N.T.) A CIRCLE,

Bend (sideways) in the pose of aiming (an arrow) at an eagle. This sentence expresses the gesture of shooting an eagle.

OR RAISE YOUR WAIST AND YOUR BACK,

Here is another method. Lie down face up and prop the back of both hands against the floor to raise your waist; draw in your feet and touch the ground with your head.

LIKE A HALF MOON.

This is the method of raising your waist.

CROSS YOUR FINGERS BEHIND YOUR HEAD

This is another method. Cross the ten fingers of both hands behind your head to hug the jade pillow (the occiput, N.T.)

AND TWIST LEFT AND RIGHT.

It is said above to cross your fingers behind your head. Next, turn your head (and the whole upper torso, N.T.) twisting now left and now right.

THE BREATH IN THE HANDS AND THE BACK IS STRONG AND FULL,

This means: when guiding and leading (the breath), straighten strongly both hands so as to urge on the Original Breath.

(AND) IT EXITS FROM THE TIP OF YOUR FINGERS.

It is said above that when your hands are strongly stretched, the Original Breath is full and exits naturally from the tips of the ten fingers.

SHAKE AND PULL THE FOUR LIMBS,

Here it means that when guiding and leading (the breath), you must shake, pull and move your hands and feet. It speaks, therefore, of the four limbs.

FIRMLY SEIZE THE THREE PASSES,

Here it says that when guiding and leading (the breath) you should perhaps block the breath, or firmly tighten your fists, and massage your toes. The three passes are your mouth, your hands and your feet (according to the Pai Wen P'ien, the eyes, the nose, the mouth, N. T.).

THOROUGHLY MASSAGE THE ONE-FOOT HOUSE,

Use both hands to rub your face.

AS WELL AS THE SEA OF BREATH.

Massage (your lower abdomen) with both hands (as well.)

TAP YOUR TEETH TOGETHER TO GATHER THE SPIRITS,

When ingesting breath, and when guiding and leading (it), it is, in general, necessary first to tap your teeth together thirty-six times to collect the spirits of the five viscera. Teeth mean the upper and lower incisors. This is called the heavenly drum. The spirits will gather when hearing the drum roll.

CLOSE YOUR PUPILS, FORTIFY THE PASSES,

The "pupils" refer to your eyes. The passes are your mouth, hands and feet. It says to block the three passes so that the ten thousand evils will not enter.

OBSCURE THE MIND, RELAX THE BONES.

To state that ten thousand thoughts do not enter (means) to relax. "The bones" refers to the body bones. It is said here to make your mind like ashes so that the ten thousand thoughts will not enter (and) to relax the body bones to resemble the great void.

BREATHE AT WILL, (BREATHE) TO AND FRO,

Close your mouth, breathe at will through the soul's hut (the nose.) It comes and goes.

AND REALIZE THAT THE BREATH IS HARMONIZED AND EQUALIZED.

Be conscious of the harmony and evenness of the breath entering and exiting through the nose.

PRESS AND BLOCK THE THROAT PASS.

Wait for the exit of the harmonious breath into the throat, then block it to prevent the external air from entering and the internal air from exiting. This is the pressing and blocking of the throat pass.

WHEN IT IS PRESSED AND BLOCKED, THEN SWALLOW.

The previous blocking obtains the Original Breath inside the throat. When (what is) outside does not enter and (what is) inside does not exit, then swallow.

UNDERTAKE THREE CONSECUTIVE SWALLOWINGS,

This again talks about the usual method in swallowing breath. The three consecutive swallowings are (made) out of one blocked breath. Swallow three times consecutively. Do not allow the saliva and the air to be swallowed at the same time.

TURN YOUR TONGUE AROUND TO RINSE AND LET IN (THE BREATH.)

When blocking the breath, make the air exit slightly into your mouth and hold it in your mouth. Move your tongue slightly, then rinse and let in the breath.

GULP IT DOWN TO THE TAN-T'IEN.

It says here to rinse and gulp down the Original Breath straight into the TAN-T'IEN. The lower TAN-T'IEN is three inches below the navel. It is also called the sea of breath.

USE YOUR MIND TO LEAD THE BREATH,

When gulping down the breath, use your mind to lead the breath into the lower TAN-T'IEN.

WHICH MAKES THE "KU" SOUND.

When gulping breath down, there are "Ku, Ku" sounds like water dripping through a hole. These are heard distinctly.

ONE SWALLOWING (CONSISTS OF) THREE SWALLOWINGS.

It is said here that when swallowing breath, one swallowing becomes (actually) three swallowings. One blocking of the breath is then followed by three consecutive swallowings.

SWALLOW AGAIN AS BEFORE,

This means that once the three swallowings are completed, you must let the breath exit and enter at will through the soul's hut (the nose, N.T.) When the breath is harmonized, undertake three consecutive swallowings as before. This is what is called "swallow again as before."

THIRTY-SIX SWALLOWINGS.

After each three consecutive swallowings, wait for the breath to be harmonized. As before, swallow three times right away to reach thirty-six swallowings which is the constant fitness of the breath. The Yellow Court Canon says, "Thirty-six gulps into the jade pool". This is what it means. If you have not yet interrupted grains, then eat little and be sure your stomach is empty and clean. Regardless of sitting or lying down, swallow (the breath) as soon as the stomach is empty. There should be three hundred and sixty swallowings each day within the ten periods. If one has practiced ingesting for long, and reached three hundred and sixty swallowings, it is considered a medium achievement. Reaching one thousand two hundred swallowings (per day) is considered a great achievement, the utmost of the Embryonic Breath. If (one) closes the breath and counts to one thousand (counts), or one hundred breathing during the small Embryonic Breath, then this is also regarded as a great achievement. Thus, if one is unable to refine the form and transform the substance, even if one obtains the prolongation of life, one is identical to a withered tree which lacks the sap. If there is any perverse effect, sudden sickness or calamity in the practice of nourishing, one should, in general, rely only on the method of breath ingestion to seek to manage it quickly in order to achieve a difference.

When swallowing breath, it is not necessary to swallow only thirty-six (times.) (Strive) to reach thirty swallowings, (then) fifty, sixty, seventy, eighty, ninety, (and then) one hundred swallowings, so as to have the air move inside the abdomen and the breath communicate within the four limbs. Then lie down also and relax, stretch your hands (away from your body), close your mouth, and let the breath exit and enter at will through the soul's hut (the nose.) Let the breathing be subtle and then subtler, reducing it only. Take in much breath and exhale little. This is the method to achieve the genuine embryo.

THE EMBRYONIC BREATH IS (THUS) ACHIEVED.

The Embryonic Breath is the three consecutive swallowings going up to thirty-six swallowings, which is the achievement.

THE GREAT WAY (TAO) IS NON-ACTION (WU-WEI),

"The great way (TAO)" is an analogy to the human body. "Non-action (WU WEI)" is doing nothing.

When practicing the Embryonic Breath, regardless of sitting or lying down, whether walking or standing, let the breath roam in the body as if it were in the great void. That is achieving the state of NON- ACTION (WU WEI), which is (to be) as though devoid of body. When (one) achieves to be without a body, this is to be without confused thinking. When (one) is without confused thinking, then the Original Breath appears naturally without being sought after. It comes naturally without having to be coaxed.

AND (THEREFORE) IT IS ACTION INDEED.

This statement seems contrary and ruinous to the great way (TAO.) It is only because students might persist so erroneously in NON-ACTION (WU WEI) that he says, "it is action indeed."

BEING ABLE OF NON-ACTION,

This is what the previous commentary said: to let it roam in the body as if it were in the great void.

IT IS CALLED NON-THOUGHT.

This is what the previous commentary said, also: to be like the great void. What is void is without minding. This is called non-thought.

IF ONE IS ABLE OF NON-THOUGHT,

The previous commentary said if able of voidness, one is without minding. Then naturally one has no thought.

THEN THE TEN THOUSAND THINGS RETURN BY THEMSELVES.

The ten thousand things are the ten thousand people. The ten thousand people point to the return of the Original. "Return by themselves" means they return naturally. It says that if one is able to be without thought, the Original Breath returns naturally to the body. If, however, one acts to seek after this Original Breath, it is like climbing a tree in search of a fish.

THE PHENOMENON OF THE WAY IS NOT DUAL.

This means that the method of the restoration of the genuine breath has been the same since ancient times.

IT DOES NOT RELY ON ACTION.

It speaks of utter naturalness. If one acts to force it, then it is wrong.

THERE IS NO COLD AND NO HEAT,

This (describes) the merit of the restored genuine breath returning to the origin. If having practiced for long, one feels then neither cold nor heat.

NO THIRST AND NO HUNGER,

This is the effect of the genuine breath. If one has practiced industriously, then one feels neither thirst nor hunger.

(IT IS) THE WONDER OF WONDERS AND THE MOST SUBTLE OF THE SUBTLE.

The above two expressions are praising the unthinkableness of the restored Genuine Breath. (As Lao Tzu said), "It is looked at, but cannot be seen; it is listened to, but cannot be heard; it is grasped at, but cannot be held". It is the same as the "elusive", the "inaudible" and the "subtle". (From TAO TE CHING, CHAPTER 14, N.T.)

DEVOID OF ANY SENSATION AND WITHOUT DESIRES,

"Devoid of any sensation" is the flavor of no flavor, thus: constancy. It is said here that the way (TAO) is plain, and constant and without any desire.

PLEASE YOURSELF WITH THE TAO.

"Please" means "take delight in". This talks about the natural contentment achieved after man obtains the way (TAO), of restoring the Genuine Breath to the Original. His destiny is, moreover, in himself and not in the hands of heaven. After he has accomplished the merit, he can ascend to heaven in broad daylight. He can sit, stay, and stand on nothingness. A court of ten thousand souls will pay him homage. Though the high mountain may collapse, he does not (so) collapse. The world may go to pieces and he does not fall apart. Therefore, he is naturally content.

THE PERFECT MAN WHO DWELLS ON THE TAO (WAY),

This points to the people who study the way (TAO.)

SHOULD REMEMBER IT AND PAY RESPECT TO IT.

The sentence here means that the people who seek after the teaching of immortality must pay serious attention to this text, which may be carved in stone or be carried respectfully on one's body.

The end of the CHEN CH'I HUAN YÜAN MING.

CHI KO HSÜAN LAO TZU CHIEH CHIEH
AN EDITED TEXT OF KO HSÜAN'S COMMENTARY TO SELECTIONS OUT OF LAO TZU'S (TAO TE CHING)
by YEN LING FENG.[2]

Chapter 1

TAO TE CHING EXCERPTED TEXT:
In order to observe its wonder, be constantly void.

KO HSÜAN'S COMMENTARY:
This means guarding the void.

Chapter 2

A sage therefore manages all affairs through non-action.

---

[2] The complete text is taken out of the WU CH'IU PEI CHAI LAO TZU CHI CHENG. Excerpts from this commentary are found in the TAO TE CHEN CHING CHU SHU in the Tao Tsang Vol. XXII, p. 191; Harvard Yenching 404; Wieger 704.

This means being natural.

Chapter 3

Keep the people from becoming robbers.
This means that when there is no evil breath, robbers cannot enter. If one practices the One, then evil breath leaves.

Not seeing what may excite desires
This means non-action.

Keeps the mind away from disorder.
This means the constant guarding of the One.

Therefore, in a sage's government,
This means the mastering of the body.

He empties the mind and fills the abdomen.
"He empties the mind" is having no evil thoughts. "Fills the abdomen" is blocking breath and cultivating tranquillity.

Chapter 4

TAO is void, yet it is used.
"Void" means the One. It is the One which is in the body. A person should often practice it.

It will never overflow.
This means guarding nature.

It resolves tangles.
This means that there is no anger.

It is in harmony with the light.
The way (TAO) of the wise man is constantly in harmony with the spiritual light.

Chapter 7

Heaven is everlasting and earth is long enduring. The reason why heaven and earth are able to last and endure is because they do not live for themselves. They can therefore live long.
"Heaven is everlasting" means the mudball (NI WAN.) "Earth is long enduring" means (the lower) elixir field (TAN T'IEN.) The mudball goes down to the scarlet palace (CHIANG-KUNG) and the elixir field ascends to practice the One (HSING YI.) The upper and lower primordial breaths flow and meet. Hundreds of joints are immersed and moistened. The harmonious breath will be produced naturally. So is the great way (TAO) completed. It therefore says, "Live long."

Chapter 8

(The attributes of) the superior instinct resemble those of water.
"Instinct" indicates the saliva in the mouth. Rinse with it, then the sweet spring appears. Hold it and swallow it. It will go down to benefit thousands of spirits. If you want to practice this, you should often rinse the flowery pond (HUA-CH'IH) in the morning. When your mouth is full of saliva, lift up your head and swallow the saliva so as to benefit thousands of spirits and increase your vitality.

(During) speech, (this) instinct is trustworthy. This means that when vitality flows throughout the body, thousands of spirits assemble. The sweet spring in your mouth will therefore gush naturally. You can rinse with it and swallow it endlessly. If people do not know this, how could they practice this? Therefore, when the sage practices the One, how could there be no early splendor?

When in action, this instinct is timely.

This means that when a sage serves the way (TAO), he heals his body by removing evil and guile. This is to be taken later as a model by the wise. The seven (attributes of) the instinct come about because the One is circulating throughout the body benefiting thousands of spirits (the word SHAN, perfection, virtue, instinct appears seven times in this version of the eighth chapter of the TAO TE CHING - N.T.)

Chapter 9

Should you try to strike and sharpen an edge, the edge will not last long.
To strike in the upper part means to let out words. To strike in the lower part means to lose control over the vitality (the semen, N.T.) Letting out words causes discord. Losing control over vitality causes your hair to turn gray and your teeth to fall out.

When gold and jade fill your hall, you will not be able to keep them safe.
This means that breath and blood are the gold, the semen is the jade. If you practice the One, the upper and lower parts will open up to each other. There will be loud noises. Your limbs and joints will help each other. Your eyes will be bright and sparkling. These are the effects of fulfilling the One.

Arrogance with wealth and honor will bring about your downfall.
This means that those who enjoy riches and honor are mostly greedy for power and wealth. They are not willing to study the way (TAO.) They will die. When they die, they cannot retain their power and wealth. Even if they have accumulated an enormous amount of money, of what use will it be to them when they are already dead?

Chapter 10

Can you become baby-like?
This means embracing and practicing the primordial breath without toiling. The great way (TAO) flows and spreads out (with the natural grace of) a baby.

Can you be without knowledge while your intelligence reaches the four quarters?
"Reaches the four quarters" is to know the eight directions. To close your mind and block your thoughts will enable you to exist for thousands of generations. If you can practice this, you will be known to the Supreme August.

Chapter 11

The function of a vessel arises from non-being.
This means that when the ancients molded clay into a vessel, the vessel had to be fired to get rid of the water since otherwise the vessel would fail and would not become a vessel. If you want to practice the way (TAO) and (yet) do not enter a room to refine your body regularly, then you will only be an ordinary person certain to die.

Thus, practical results arise from its being.
This states the existence of the way (TAO.)

The function arises from its non-being.
This states that a sage holds the One and practices naturalness. He does not need anything else.

Chapter 12

The five colors blind men's eyes.
This does not mean that human beings are blind. You would like to see, but all you see are the black and yellow colors (of heaven and earth, N.T.) You do not see the coming and going of the divinities, their jeweled carriage and their brilliant five-colored light. This is why it says, "blind men's eyes."

The five musical sounds deafen men's ears.
This does not mean that human beings are deaf. You would like to hear, but all you can hear is the sounds of chimes and drums. You do not hear the sound of the divinities. This is why it says, "deafen men's ears."

Galloping, chasing, and hunting maddens the human mind.
This means that when a man dies, he returns to dust. His family attending the funeral, his relatives running around for the funeral, the confusion, the crying, the weeping, the burial into the grave, and the funeral procession through the fields, all of this makes the close relatives frantic and the distant ones sad. This is why it says, "maddens."

Chapter 13

Achieving it is a surprise.
This means that when the way (TAO) is achieved, thousands of spirits come along and sing in your abdomen. They meet and talk to you. When the five spirits are known, the primordial breath flows freely. This is why it says, "Achieving it is a surprise".

Losing it, is a surprise.
This means that once the breath is lost and the sperm is spent, the vitality is depleted and as a consequence, the One is lost. Your hair will turn gray, your teeth will fall out and you will die. The cries from people's grief rise to the sky and the lamentations of the souls startle the divinities in heaven. This is why it says, "Losing it, is a surprise."

If I had no body, what calamity could come to me?
To be oblivious of the body and to nourish the vitality is called "had no body".

Chapter 14

Being unceasing and continuous, it cannot be defined.
This means the way (TAO) enters your skin, bones, and joints. It says, therefore, that "being unceasing and continuous, it cannot be defined".

Chapter 17

When the highest supreme exists, those who are lower know its existence.
This means that it is known that the mudball (NI-WAN) is in the upper part and the elixir field (TAN T'IEN) in the lower part. The male and the female meet in the scarlet palace (CHIANG-KUNG.) Closing the mind and holding your fists tight will make the primordial breath flow and circulate. Your ears will hear divine sounds. You know that in the lower part there is the noise in the abdomen. When you practice the One, there will be the music of the chimes and the drums.

Next, they would get close and praise.
"Getting close" refers to the superior souls, "praising" to the inferior souls.

Chapter 20

Renounce learning and anxiety will end.
This means that you should do away with canons and books and practice the One.

The life force is latent in darkness and unfathomable.
This means that the Primordial Breath is transformed into life force.

Life force is of the essence. In it is the evidence.
This refers to the semen. The perfect man is the one whose semen does not transform and blood does not hide. He

practices the One in his body which therefore (appears or) is the evidence.

Its name has never vanished from ancient times up to now.
"Name" refers to the way (TAO.) The sage never dies. His name lives forever.

Chapter 22

Abundance causes perplexity.

This means that ordinary people have many thoughts and desires. They have no confidence in themselves. Therefore, they are perplexed.

The sage therefore embraces the One and becomes a model to the world.
This means it is good to remember the One and practice the way (TAO) and hold it in the body.

Chapter 25

Revolving (it) without being weary
This means that the sage practices the One in his body. It flows and circulates through his four limbs, hundreds of joints, nine orifices and hundreds of channels. This is why it says, "revolving (it) without being weary".

May be regarded as the mother of the world.
This means that guarding the way (TAO) so as to hold on to the One is the mother of the world.

Within the realm, there are four that are great. The king is one of them.

This means that the lungs are great, the heart is great, the liver is great, and the spleen is great. The water of the kidneys produces the One and the king dwells in the One. This means that the breath of the spleen rules over the four directions. That is the practice of the One.

Chapter 26

(How can a ruler) regard the body lightly in the world?
This means treating death lightly. Even a man as noble as a king should hold the One to prolong life. To see this but not to learn from it is taking the body lightly. When he dies, even though he may have jade and gold engravings, how could they benefit his body?

Hastiness destroys self-mastery.
This means that he who is hasty cannot live long.

Chapter 27

He who closes well needs no bolts, yet it (the door, N.T.) cannot be opened.
This refers to the blocking of the breath and holding the fists tight. The heavenly female is being locked in the upper part, the earthly male is being locked in the lower part. This is why it says, "needs no bolts".

An able binder needs no rope, yet his knot cannot be untied.
This indicates binding and holding the souls. The sage embraces the superior souls and holds the inferior souls. This is why it says, "cannot be untied".

Chapter 28

Being aware of maleness, yet keeping to femaleness is being the gorge (repository) of the world.

"Maleness" refers to the superior souls, "femaleness" refers to the inferior souls. This means that the spirits come and go inside the body. He who practices the One therefore imitates and guards the nature, holds the fists tight, and blocks off the breath to embrace and hold the souls.

Being the gorge of the world, you are able to retain the constant virtue and return to infancy.
"The gorge" is the mouth. This means to practice the One and block the breath. Following profoundly non-action will prevent you from aging. You will return to infancy.

Being a model to the world is having constant unerring virtue,
This means that the way (TAO) is for the immortal to practice the One so as to be a model to the world.

Returning to infinity,
"Infinity" means constantly sustaining life and practicing the One.

(And) returning to the natural uncarved block.
This means retaining naturalness.

Chapter 30

To assist a ruler by upholding the way (TAO) is not to make use of arms to conquer the world.
This refers to the mouth as the use of the force of arms. A slip of the tongue causes the use of the force of arms. Vitality (the sperm, N.T.) will leap and bound and the upper and lower souls will infringe upon each other. Then the spirits will be disturbed and leave the body.

These matters will certainly earn their due back.
This means that if, when you practice the One, your mind is peaceful and your will calm, the spirits will return to your body.

Chapter 31

Sharp weapons are instruments of bad omen.
The expression "instruments of bad omen" refers to those who, because they talk heedlessly, will lose their live body. When the body is endangered, the instruments are destroyed as well.

They are not the instruments of a superior man.
This means that the mouth brings about discussions and thus causes use of the force of arms. When the Yin (ejaculation, N.T.) is strong, its ax will kill the body, thus being "the instruments of bad omen."

Chapter 33

He who behaves strongly, has a firm will.
This means that the way (TAO) is to be practiced day and night without any break.

He who does not lose his place, endures.
This means that the One is not lost.

He who dies yet does not perish has longevity.
This means that to experience "deliverance from the corpse" (SHIH CHIEH, see Glossary), is to be reborn after death.

Chapter 39

Having attained the One, the heavens are purified.
This means that the mudball (NI WAN) is in a person's head, wherefrom the fresh and pure breath descends. This is why it is said, "are purified".

Having attained the One, the earth is peaceful.
This means that when there is no licentiousness in the elixir field (TAN T'IEN), the vitality will reside in the body. It is said, therefore, "peaceful".

Having attained the One, the spirit is magically responsive.
"The spirit" is the mind. The mind is divinely magical, it is the lord of the five viscera. This is why it says "magically responsive."

Having attained the One, the valley is full.
"The valley" is the mouth which is the palace of the flowery pond that can bring about the sweet spring. Therefore, it is said, "full".

Having attained the One, thousands of entities are alive.
This means that thousands of entities are different in form, yet they all share in the possession of the One in order to live. This is why it is said, "alive".

Having attained the One, the nobles and the king are rectified.
This indicates the spleen which is in the middle, in order to control the four directions. It is said, therefore, "are rectified".

The One brings about all of these.
This means that heaven and earth, man, spirit, water, spring, and thousands of entities all share in the One in order to live. This is why it is said, "The One brings about all of these things".

Without clarity, heaven might disintegrate.
This says that if the mudball (NI WAN) does not attain the One, the brain will wither, the hair will gray, and the teeth will fall out. It says, therefore, "disintegrate".

Without tranquillity, the earth might be agitated.
This means that if the elixir field (TAN T'IEN) does not attain

the One, then vitality will dissipate. It says, therefore, "might be agitated".

Without magical responsiveness, the spirit might end.
This means that if the mind is disorderly, the body is empty and ages fast. It says, therefore, "might end".

Without being filled, the valley might be parched.
This means that when the mouth loses the One, the flowery pond does not produce saliva. It says, therefore, "parched".

Nobility must, therefore, have its origin in humbleness.
This means that if a man seeks longevity, he should regard the Primordial Breath as (his) mother. This is why it says, "origin".

The high must have the low as its foundation.
This means that a person practicing the way (TAO) should regard the elixir field of primordial importance for nurturing his vitality and strengthening his brain. Therefore, it says, "as its foundation".

Therefore, the highest renown is without renown.
This means that the way (TAO) is the original truth.
It is nameless. Embrace the One and hold (it) inside.
Do not seek it from outside. This is why it says, "without renown".

Chapter 41

Making a big vessel takes long.
This means that holding the One without weariness helps to attain the way (TAO) in old age.

Chapter 45

Keeping still, overcomes heat.

"Keeping still, overcomes heat" means that non-action insures the spirit to hold the One.

Being pure and calm is the right model to the world.
This means that going into a remote mountain to practice keeping pure in order to guard nature will make you become a perfect man.

Chapter 49

Regard the mind of hundreds of surnames (the people) as your own mind.
This means that when you know the way (TAO) and practice breathing, by holding the spirit as the mind, your breath will flow and spread to hundreds of joints which have hundreds of spirits with hundreds of different names sharing a dwelling in your body. It says, therefore, "regard other people's mind as your own mind".

Then goodness is attained.
This means that when you practice the One to nurture the spirit, the spirit will be harmonious and the form pliant. Evil will vanish and only what is right and good will be left. Your bones will be strong and your marrow genuine. This is why it says, "goodness is attained".

Faith is attained.
This means that if man has faith in the One, then the One also has faith in man. If man has no faith in the One, then the One is produced according to man. Therefore, the way (TAO) constantly comprises faith.

Chapter 50

In him (a sage), there is no place for death.

This means that a sage embraces the spirit, holds the One, practices breathing and holds his fists tight to do the Embryonic Breathing. The principle (TAO) that nothing can hurt is in his mind and the Genuine Breath is present. There is, therefore, no place for destruction.

Chapter 53

If I had great knowledge, I would walk on the great way (TAO.)
Day and night, I would be most anxious to think of and hold the One in my body.

Yet people like the small by-paths.
This means that people like what is evil and false. They walk on the wrong byways.

The field is filled with weeds.
This means that man does not cultivate the One. Day and night he improves his (exterior) appearance (by eating grains, N.T.) so he fails and becomes ill. His mind is, therefore, ill-cultivated.

The granaries are quite empty.
This means that if man does not hold and strengthen the One, his five viscera will be empty. It says, therefore, "empty".

Carrying sharp swords,
This means that if a man likes to dress up in beautiful clothes, the One will leave and evil will come in. Carrying sharp swords and relying on weapons is what devils cause harm with.

And having a superabundance of wealth is called brigandage and boastfulness.
This means that if a man likes good food to improve his appearance, the One will leave him. Hundreds of diseases

will then appear. His wealth will be used towards (his) death and funeral.

This is not the way (TAO.)
This means that such a man does not practice the One. If a man thinks only of fine clothes and delicacies, he may become a robber. He cannot prevent the illness nor remove death. Therefore, that is not the way (TAO.)

Chapter 54

What is firmly planted cannot be pulled out.
This means that an expert or a superior man, who is skillful in building up his body and (his) mind through the virtues of the way (TAO), has neither virtues to show off nor feats for which to be glorified. Then his building is deeply rooted and firmly established. It cannot be uprooted by any whim of right and wrong and likes or dislikes. If the building (the body, N.T.) is made only so that he may boast with virtues, seek fame, show off merits or expect rewards, then after its beauty and virtue are displayed, its hidden merit is still not accomplished.

Eventually, it will be uprooted by the impermanence and hindrance of its past destiny. Therefore, Huai Nan Tzu said, "Though the appearance of a building is splendid and strong, it can still be destroyed by a fire. Though fire is hot, it may be extinguished by water. Though water flows, it may be stopped by earth. Though wood is strong, it may be cut by an ax. Therefore, only he who can build what is not a (physical) building, will not be uprooted."

Chapter 56

Those who know do not speak,
This means the One is indescribable.

(And) those who speak do not know.
This means that those who talk do not know the One.

Block the aperture, close the doors.
This means one is to close off the nine orifices, protect the life force and hold the breath.

Chapter 57

Rule a nation through proper and correct measure. When using arms, practice surprise.
This means that those who nourish the body should be right in their mind. They should not hurt themselves by the arms of the mouth. "A nation" refers to the body.

The more prohibitions there are in the world, the poorer the people become.
This means having action.

Therefore, a sage says, "I will do nothing and the people will be transformed by themselves.
This means that guarding nature will ensure the flowing and circulation of the Primordial Breath.

"I will deal in no business and the people become rich by themselves.
This means that when a person does not deal in business, his form, breath, vitality, blood, and channels will naturally be full.

"When I like quietude, the people will be proper and correct by themselves.
This means that when a person is humble without any evil thought, the breath will stay in his body.

"When I have no desires, the people will naturally be simple and honest".

This means that when a person has no lust or desire and holds firmly the One, then his vitality will be pure and strong because it has not been weakened and wasted.

Chapter 58

The good become evil again.
This means that having attained the blessings of the way (TAO), if a man cannot hold the One, usually he would be arrogant and evil thoughts will reappear.

The delusions of the people have subsisted for a long time.
This means that the worldly people cannot hold the One. They are deceived by what is evil and false. They lose blessings and incur calamities. It has been this way for a very long time. It is not something that is just happening now.

Therefore, a sage is square but not sharply edged,
"Square" means the correct and the proper way of the One. You should hold it and practice it firmly. You should promise yourself not to be harmed again by self-imposed evil.

Sharp and clean but not cutting,
"Sharp and clean" indicates the purity of the breath. One should not harm the practice of the way (TAO) with dirtiness and turbidity.

Straight but not reckless,
This means that the merit of the One is smooth yet it yields and bends with the mind. It does not have the criterion of straightness as a carpenter's inked lines.

Bright but not dazzling.
"Bright" indicates that the spirits are bright and they flow freely to moisten the inside of the body. You do not need to light up a candle.

Chapter 59

Early serving is the repeated accumulation of the attributes (TE) of the way (TAO).
This means that the reason why all the evil goes to hide is because of the accumulated breath from the repeated practice of the One.

Because of the repeated accumulation of the attributes (TE), there is nothing that cannot be overcome.
This means that when the One is practiced repeatedly and breath is accumulated, evil will be expelled and illnesses will be cured. Therefore there is nothing that cannot be overcome.

When nothing cannot be overcome, one does not know what is its limit.
This means that when the One circulates in the body, it expels what is evil and cures diseases. What is its limit is unknown. Therefore, one will have a long life.

Chapter 60

It is not that the evil spirits have lost their magical powers. It is that their magical power does not harm the people.
It does not mean that the evil spirits have no magical powers. It is because the way (TAO) resides in people's bodies, therefore, the evil powers cannot harm the people.

Not only their magical power does not harm the people, a ruling sage also does not harm the people.
This means that when a person practices the way (TAO), he is identical to a divinity. Internally, he has no hidden faults. Therefore, the evil spirits cannot do harm to him. Externally, he has no open crimes. Therefore, the ruling sages cannot punish him. When a person practices the One, the heavenly spirits protect his body externally and take care of his form internally. His primordial breath is massive only because of his practices of nourishing his own body. He follows the

heaven above. On his head, he wears the illuminating sun and moon. All the stars and constellations are inside him. Through his breathing, he has vitality and he dines on the jade flower (YÜ YING.)

Chapter 61

A big nation is like a downflowing region. It is the crossroads point of the world.
The mudball (NI WAN) is the big nation. The mouth is the small nation. The mouth receives from above and irrigates the elixir field (TAN T'IEN) below. The elixir field is the open land.

Through being subservient, a small nation gathers from a big nation.
This means that the mudball (NI WAN) resides above. It is the big nation. The elixir field (TAN T'IEN) is down below. It is the small nation. The way to practice the One is to block off the breath and swallow the saliva to have it flow down to the elixir field. The saliva is transformed into blood. The blood is transformed into semen or life force which in turn is transformed into breath. Then the Embryonic Breathing will guide it to restore and strengthen the brain. It is pushed and guided to spread widely to cover the four seas (everywhere). Therefore, the upper part takes and the lower part gathers. The small nation abases itself and is content with its lot to be gentle. It nestles in the big nation and admires and envies the latter's charm and chivalry.

Both get what they desire. Therefore, a big nation must place itself low.
"Both" indicates the mudball (NI WAN) and the elixir field (TAN T'IEN). The mudball wants the breath to ascend and the elixir field wants the breath to descend. They achieve the one spirit together.

Chapter 63

Practice non-action.
This means that, he who practices the One does not do it consciously for the body.

Serve no affairs.
This means that, he who serves the One does not serve (outside) people.

He who promises lightly will inspire little confidence.
This means that, he who promises lightly will lose the sincerity of his self-respect.

He who knows these two principles also finds in them his model and rule.
This means that, when one abandons knowledge and guards simplicity, illnesses will be expelled and the breath will prosper. This is the model and rule by which to treat the body.

It is opposite to things.
This means that the profundity of the One lies in the descending of the supreme clarity (T'AI CH'ING) to the scarlet palace (CHIANG-KUNG). In all the forms, all things wither and die. Only you have long life. Therefore, it is the opposite to the principle of passing away and of transformation.

Chapter 67

The three entail not to venture to be the first in the world.
This means that, one should appreciate and store the life force, breath and spirit in the body so that one can prolong life.

Chapter 68

An able fighter does not lose his temper.
This means that, when a person closes his mouth and harmonizes his life force, the thousands of spirits will be delighted.

A great conqueror does not fight.
This means that when a person practices the One with his mouth, thousands of evil spirits will surrender by themselves. It therefore says, "does not fight".

Chapter 69

I dare not be the host. I would rather be the guest.
The weapon above is the mouth; the weapon below is the sex organ. When the mouth speaks recklessly, one will bring harm to oneself. Therefore, one should be humble with words. When one uses the genitals recklessly, the semen will be lost. Therefore, one dare not be a leading singer but a follower, in harmony.

Bare no arms.
Baring the arms is to show rage. An able fighter does not lose his temper. Therefore, it is as if there were no arms to bare.

There is no catastrophe greater than underestimating the enemy.
This means that he who indulges himself in intercourse will have the calamity of dying.

Underestimating the enemy is almost as bad as losing one's treasure.
"Treasure" indicates the vitality (sperm, N.T.). When one underestimates the enemy and fights often, one will lose the vital spirit.

Chapter 70

Therefore, a sage wears coarse clothes while carrying jade in his bosom.
This means that a sage values the attributes (TE) of the way TAO) and scorns forms. He wears the hide with hair, yet he embraces the One and the Primordial. He does not covet high positions. Internally, he nurtures a bright spirit. He regards the semen or life force as the jade and the breath as the gold. Wherefore, he can be transformed and ascend to the purple palace (TZU-KUNG.)

Chapter 71

He who does not know but pretends to know is sick.
This refers to people who do not understand the way (TAO). They only understand worldly business. They do not know to ingest breath, but (know) to eat delicacies. Therefore, they are sick.

Chapter 72

Do not cramp your dwelling place.
This means that one should not dwell in a narrow worldly place. The high mountains and the wide swamps are good places for cultivating the inborn nature.

Do not dislike what life depends upon.
This means that he who dislikes life, dies. Therefore, he should practice the One. He should cherish the breath and carefully protect the semen. They are the treasures of life.

Chapter 73

He who is eager in daring will be killed.
This means that if a person is given to sexual pleasures, he goes alive but returns dead. This is called "eager". If a person despises the way (TAO) and scorns the spirits, he

brings death upon himself. This is called "daring." Both mean suicide.

Therefore, even a sage regards it as difficult.
This means that nature detests eagerness in daring. It cherishes timidity and feebleness. He who knows to embrace life and to cherish breath knows the will of nature.

The way (TAO) of heaven is most able to conquer without strife.
This means that the way (TAO) of heaven cherishes harmony.

Chapter 74

Why threaten them with death?
This means that people do not seek longevity. They only seek pleasure and lust. When they hear of good, they do not cultivate it. They know evil, yet will not change. What benefit is their knowing?

An executioner is always set to execute.
This implies the mouth. On the left side of the mouth is (the Spirit named) Ssu Yin, the director of the secret. On the right side of the mouth is (the Spirit named) Ssu-Sha, the executioner. When a person has secret faults, Ssu Yin reports them to heaven to investigate his superior and inferior souls. When a person has bad and evil words, the executioner will report them to (the Spirit called) Ssu Ming, the arbiter of destiny. The arbiter will record them. When there are enough transgressions, then the person will be executed.

To take the place of the executioner so as to kill is like hewing for a master carpenter.
This means that the heavenly way (TAO) rewards good and punishes evil. In nourishing a person's body, it is like a master carpenter's working on his craft. The good will succeed, the bad will fail.

Those who take the place of the master carpenter seldom do not have their hands injured.
This implies that when people nourish their body, everyone is different in his own capacity of being good or bad. It is like the different degrees of skillfulness of individual craftsmen. The skillful will succeed in making their work. The unskilled seldom do not injure themselves.

Chapter 75

The people suffer from hunger because their ruler taxes too much in grain.
"Hunger" indicates the insufficiency of breath. The insufficiency is caused by the mouth's leisurely addiction to delicacies (made out of grains, N.T.). Much ingestion is called solidifying. Accumulation is for seclusion. Therefore, hundreds of (evil) matters are prevented.

Therefore, it is difficult to rule.
The people (with their) hundreds of surnames, indicate the hundreds of (body) channels. The reason why they are increasing and decreasing and not peaceful is because the mouth does not hold the One. Then the lips are dry and the saliva is exhausted. Therefore, the channels are lost and the life force leaks out.

People underestimate death because they seek to make a rich living.
This means that the reason why people neglect their death is because they want to nurture their forms richly so they indulge in eating. Thus, they lose the way to life. Therefore, they die.

Only those who do not stress on life are able to exalt life.
This means that if people are able to care about life when life has not yet been produced, and care about form when the form has not yet been shaped, and if people are able to think about

non-action and dwell on nature only, they are the ones to exalt the way (TAO) and a peaceful life.

Chapter 76

Therefore, when the weaponry is strong, it will not be victorious.
"Weaponry" is the mouth. When the mouth is sharp and strong, a person will be exhausted by others. When the sex organ is strong, males are harmed by females.

The strong and the big dwell below and the flexible and weak dwell above.
This implies that the hair, flexible and weak, is worn on the head by man. The body and the bones, firm and strong are made in man to labor.

Chapter 78

There is nothing in the world weaker and more flexible than water, yet none is superior to it in overcoming what is hard.
"Water" internally is the saliva in the mouth. When rinsed and swallowed, it can attack evil and destroy what is wicked. When it penetrates to the bones and marrow, it acts like fermenting yeast destroying rice. None of any (medical) prescriptions would be able to take precedence over it.

No one can practice it.
This means that the people, by holding the life force and swallowing (sometimes) the breath, do govern the blood and the hundreds of channels. (So) they use this method daily without knowing of it.

He who can accept a nation's dirtiness (should be) the ruler of the gods of the soil and the grains.

This means that in a man's (bodily) form, the left soul is the god of the earth and the right soul is the god of the grains. (A man) should manage the One Breath (which is their ruler) in order to be a ruler.

He who can accept a nation's misfortune is the king of the world.
"Nation" is the (bodily) form. This indicates that the One comes and goes in the spleen to transform the sediment and the liquid and to remove the old and to receive the new in order to nourish the five spirits (of the five viscera, N.T.) Therefore, it is the king of the viscera and the receptacles.

Right words seem to mean the opposite.
This indicates that common people want to respect what is fresh and clean. They value what is fragrant and beautiful, yet the way (TAO) makes the person who accepts what is dirty as the ruler and makes the person who deals with what is inferior as the king. This means that the One is the opposite of what common people (think).

Chapter 79

How can this be regarded as good?
This implies the mouth. This means that when there is a leading singer, others will join in. When a person is able to practice the way (TAO), the way will come and answer him. When the leading singer sings about good, good ensues. Then there will be no more grievances. Nowadays, people like to practice evil thoughts. Therefore, evil thoughts follow. They summon evil spirits which hence respond. When a leading singer sings of evil, evil ensues. How can this be good?

Therefore, a sage holds the left tally and does not demand from others.
"The left tally" is referring to the virtues of the Yang (force). This means that a sage does not settle (external) great grievances and leaves behind evoked grudges. He cultivates

the attributes (TE) of the way (TAO) by himself and does not make demands upon others.

He who has the attributes (TE) of the way (TAO) takes charge of the tallies, while he who does not have the attributes (TE) of the way (TAO) takes charge of exaction.
This means that when a person practices the attributes of the way (TAO), the arbiter of destiny (Ssu-Ming) will bestow a longer life on him. When a person practices evil, the executioner (Ssu-Sha) will confiscate what he has. This is what it means.

Chapter 80

It is ideal to have a small nation with a small population. Even if there are tens and hundreds of tools, they belong to the people, and they should not be worn out.
"A small nation" implies the body. "Tens and hundreds" implies the five viscera. The heart and the kidneys are the "tens" and the liver and the lungs are the "hundreds". When a person closes the mouth and circulates the breath, tens and hundreds of breaths are profuse. None is not in use.

Let the people return to the use of tying ropes.
This means that when a person has the way (TAO), his breath will naturally flow and circulate for the use of the body, just like the tokens of knotted rope.

Savor the food and enjoy the beautiful clothing.
This implies that a person will find relish in ingesting breath and enjoying the way (TAO) as (his) beautiful clothing.

Be happy in the culture.
This means that a person is happy with the body and the spirit. He embraces (his) abdomen and it sings.

Though the neighboring nations are within sight and the dog's barkings and the rooster's crowings within earshot, the people will never exchange visits up to their old age.
"The neighboring nations" are the two ears. The two ears are within sight of each other in order to guard peace. They make the spirit and the breath guard their own places. They do not visit or bother each other. Therefore, a person is able to keep his hearing clear up to his old age.

Chapter 81

Honest words are not beautiful. Beautiful words are not honest.
This means that he who believes in the words of the way (TAO) does not extol worldly affairs. He who extols worldly affairs will not believe in the words of the way (TAO).

ERRATA

Read:

Page 155
Five Elements (Wu-**H**sing)

Five Notes (Wu-**Y**in).

Page 161
P'eng Ch**ü**

Page 168
Yin Tan Pai Y**ü**

Yü-Lu 玉廬

GLOSSARY

Animals (The Astrological)
One animal assigned to each of the 12 earthly branches: 1. **Tzu:** Rat, 2. **Ch'ou:** Ox, 3. **Yin:** Tiger, 4. **Mao:** Rabbit, 5. **Ch'en:** Dragon, 6. **Ssu:** Snake, 7. **Wu:** Horse, 8. **Wei:** Goat, 9. **Shen:** Monkey, 10. **You:** Chicken 11. **Hsü:** Dog, 12. **Hai:** Hog.

Beat The Heavenly Drum
See Ming T'ien-Ku.

Black Warrior (Hsüan-Wu) 玄武
The seven constellations in the north. North: A symbolic name for kidneys.

Central Palace
The Abdomen.

Chang Tao-Ling 張道陵
34-156 A.D., founder of the main Taoist sect: the Cheng-Yi Sect. He is also called Chang T'ien-Shih (Celestial Master Chang.)

Ch'i 氣
It is variously translated as breath, energy, or vitality.

Ch'i-Shang 七傷
The Seven Injuries: 1. Over-fullness injures the spleen; 2. Great rage injures the liver; 3. Fatigue and dampness injure the kidneys; 4. Cold food or drink injure the lungs; 5. Grief injures the heart; 6. Storms and extreme climate injure the body; 7. Fear and indulgence injure the will.

Ch'ien 乾
    Heaven, Male, or the Sun.

Ch'i-Hai 氣海
    See Sea of Breath.

Chiang-Kung 絳宮
    See Scarlet Palace.

Ch'ih-Chai 尺宅
    The foot-long residence: the face.

Ching 精
    It is translated variously as essence, sperm or vitality.

Ch'ing-Ku 青姑
    See Corpses

Ching Men 精門
    The door of the essence or the lower Tan-T'ien.

Chiu Chung 鳩中
    The lower abdomen.

Chiu T'ou 鳩頭
    The upper collector. It may refer to the upper cooking vessel which is the esophagus.

Chu-Ch'üeh 朱雀
    See Vermilion Sparrow.

Chu-Niao 朱鳥
    See Vermilion Bird.

Ch'ui$_1$ 吹
    One of the six methods of exhalation. It belongs to the kidneys. See T'AI-HSI MI YAO KO CHÜEH. Detailed explanations given by MASPERO regarding

the six methods of exhalations are reproduced in the Preface to THE PRIMORDIAL BREATH volume II.

Chung-Kung 中宮
　　The Central Palace, the abdomen; identical with the Yellow Court which is governed by the spleen.

Cinnabar (or) Elixir Field (Tan-T'ien)
　　See Tan-T'ien.

Cloud Practice (Yün-Hsing)
　　It is a technical name for three consecutive swallowings of the breath about to be exhaled.

Cooking Vessels (The Three) (San-Chiao)
　　Esophagus, interior stomach canal and the bladder canal.

Corpses (The Three) (San-Shih)
　　Also referred to as San-Ku (The three poisons) or San Ch'ung (The three worms). They are the three ferocious and ill-intentioned demons situated in each of the three elixir fields (Tan-T'ien). The top one is called P'eng-Chü or Ch'ing-Ku, the middle one is called P'eng-Chih or Pai-Ku, the lower one is called P'eng-Chiao or Hsüeh-Ku.

Creatures (Thirty-Six) (San-Shih-Liu Ch'in)
　　Three creatures assigned to each of the twelve earthly branches: 1. **Tzu:** swallow, rat, bat; 2. **Ch'ou:** ox, crab, turtle; 3. **Yin:** fox, leopard, tiger; 4. **Mao:** hedgehog, rabbit, badger; 5. **Ch'en:** dragon, crocodile-dragon, fish; 6. **Ssu:** eel, earthworm, snake; 7. **Wu:** deer, roebuck, horse; 8. **Wei:** goat, eagle, wild goose; 9. **Shen:** cat, ape, monkey; 10. **You:** pheasant, chicken, crow; 11. **Hsü:** dog, wolf, jackal; 12. **Hai:** pig, great lizard, hog.

Dark Female (Hsüan-P'in)
Also translated as "mysterious female". A name for the alchemical womb where the Embryo or the Embryonic Breath is being conceived.

Deliverance From The Corpse (Shih-Chieh)
A Taoist belief that immortals would appear to be dead and allow their body to be interred, yet the body would disappear from the tomb after burial and ascend to heavens.

Door Of The Essence (Ching-Men)
Lower Tan-T'ien.

Door Of Heaven (T'ien-Men)
The nose

Elixir (Tan)
The accomplished Embryonic Breath. It is generally believed as the elixir pill for immortality.

Embryo (T'ai)
The coagulated or gathered energy from the revolving mixture of the external and the internal air in the lower Tan-T'ien.

Embryonic Breath (T'ai-Hsi)
Air or energy coagulated or gathered in the lower Tan-T'ien. If obtained, it allows the practitioner to stop usual breathing for an extended period of time.

Erh Ching 二景
Two views: the external and the internal views. Also translated as two images. The sun and the moon.

Fifth Night Watch (Wu-ching, Wu-keng)
About 4 A.M. The period from night-fall to day break was divided into five watches. It is also called the fifth drum (Wu-Ku) or the fifth night-period (Wu-Ye).

Five Colors (Wu-Sse)
Black, corresponding with water; Red, corresponding with fire; Green, corresponding with wood; White, corresponding with metal; yellow corresponding with earth.

Five Diseases (Wu-Lao)
The diseases caused by over-exertion of the five viscera.

Five Elements (Wu-hsing)
Earth, metal, water, wood, and fire.

Five Grains (Wu-Ku)
Lists Vary. They are generally grains of all sorts. Wheat, barley, millet, sorghum, and rice; Rice, millet, wheat, oats, pulse; Sesame, millet of two kinds, wheat, pulse.

Five Notes (Wu-yin)
The five notes of the Chinese musical scale: Kung, Shang, Chiao, Chih, Yü. They are the do, re, mi, sol, la.

Five Sacred Mountains (Wu-Yüeh)
The East Mountain or T'ai-Shan in Shan-Tung; the West Mountain or Hua-Shan in Shen-Hsi; the South Mountain or Heng-Shan in Hu-Nan; the North Mountain or Heng-Shan in Ho-Pei; and the Middle Mountain or Sung-Shan in Ho-Nan. They symbolize probably the five viscera.

Five Viscera (Wu-Tsang)
They are: the heart, corresponding to fire; the lungs, corresponding to metal; the liver, corresponding to

wood; the kidneys, corresponding to water; and the spleen, corresponding to earth.

Flavors (The Five) (Wu-Wei)
Sweet, sour, bitter, pungent, and salty.

Flowery Pond (Hua-Ch'ih)
The mouth.

Foot Long Residence
The face.

Germs (The Five Internal Grains) (Wu-Ya)
The five genuine breaths of the five elements corresponding to the five viscera.

Grand Ultimate (T'ai-Chi)
The primordial chaos, the state when the heaven and the earth were not separated yet. It is also called T'ai-Ch'u (The Grand Beginning) or T'ai-Yi (The Ultimate One). It refers to the Absolute, the Great Tao.

Granting of the Rain (Yü-Shih)
A swallowing of the breath with the saliva.

Gushing Spring
See Yüng-Ch'üan.

Ho$_1$ 呵
One of the six methods of exhalation. It belongs to the heart. See T'AI-HSI MI YAO KO CHÜEH. Detailed explanations given by MASPERO regarding the six methods of exhalations are reproduced in the Preface to THE PRIMORDIAL BREATH, volume II.

Hsi$_1$ 嘻
One of the six methods of exhalation. It belongs to the three cooking vessels. See T'AI-HSI MI YAO KO

CHÜEH. Detailed explanations given by MASPERO regarding the six methods of exhalations are reproduced in the Preface to THE PRIMORDIAL BREATH volume II.

Hsi$_4$ 呬

One of the six methods of exhalation. It belongs to the lungs. See T'AI-HSI MI YAO KO CHÜEH. Detailed explanations given by MASPERO regarding the six methods of exhalations are reproduced in the Preface to THE PRIMORDIAL BREATH volume II.

Hsü$_1$ 嘘

One of the six methods of exhalation. It belongs to the liver. See T'AI-HSI MI YAO KO CHÜEH. Detailed explanations given by MASPERO regarding the six methods of exhalations are reproduced in the Preface to THE PRIMORDIAL BREATH volume II.

Hsüan-P'in 玄牝

See Dark Female.

Hsüeh-Ku 血姑

See Corpses.

Hu$_1$ 呼

One of the six methods of exhalation. It belongs to the spleen. See T'AI-HSI MI YAO KO CHÜEH. Detailed explanations given by MASPERO regarding the six methods of exhalations are reproduced in the Preface to THE PRIMORDIAL BREATH volume II.

Hua-Ch'ih 華池

The mouth.

Huang-Ning 黃寧

The state attained after one has successfully practiced with the Yellow Court Canon.

Huang-T'ing-Ching 黃庭經
See Yellow Court Canon.

Hun 魂
The three superior souls of the human body. They are named: T'ai-Kuang (Embryonic Light), Shuang-Ling (Pleasant Magic) and You-Ching (Remote Spirit).

Hun-Tun 混沌
Primordial chaos, also called "uncarved block" by Chuang Tzu.

Jade Flower (Yü-Ying)
Saliva.

Jade Juice (Yü-Yeh)
Saliva.

Jade Pond (Yü-Ch'ih)
The mouth.

Jade Spring (Yü-Ch'üan)
Saliva.

Ko Hsüan 葛玄
244-325 A.D., sobriquet (Tzu) Hsiao-Hsien. He was born in Chü-Jung of Tan-Yang (near Nanking). Since he was young, he had liked the Taoist practices. He studied alchemy, refining of the breath, healing diseases, and nurturing life from Tso Yüan-Fang. He traveled many famous mountains, such as Kua-Ts'ang, Nan-Yüeh, Lo-Fu and T'ien-T'ai. He taught and practiced Taoist healing and nurturing. Among his famous students are Chang T'ai-Yen, K'ung Lung, and Cheng Ssu-Yüan. His writings include A Preface to Tao-Te-Ching, Ch'ing-Ching-Ching, Tuan-Ku-Shih-Fang, and Ju-Shan-Ching-Ssu-Ching. Lao Tzu Chieh Chieh was attributed to him by some Taoists. He was

regarded as an immortal and was called Ko Hsien-Ong or T'ai-Chi Hsien-Ong.

Ko Hung 葛洪

280-340 A.D., sobriquet (Tzu) Chih-Ch'uan, style Pao P'u-Tzu. He was born in Chü-Jung of Tan-Yang (near Nanking). Ko Hsüan was his grand uncle. Cheng Ssu-Yüan, a student of Ko Hsüan, was his teacher. He did his alchemy at Lo-Fu Mountain. After he died, he was considered as an immortal through deliverance from the corpse. His writings include Pao-P'u-Tzu and Biographies of the Immortals.

K'un 坤

Earth, Female, or the Moon.

Ling-Chih 靈芝

Also translated as magic fungus. See Mushroom of Immortality.

Ling-Yeh 靈液 **(The Magic Juice)**

Saliva.

Liu-Fu 六腑

See Receptacles.

Magic Juice (Ling-Yeh)

Saliva.

Ming T'ien-Ku 鳴天鼓

Beat the heavenly drum. A practice of covering both ears with both hands and hit the occiput with both middle fingers to make noise. Tapping of the upper and lower teeth together is also called Ming T'ien-Ku.

Mudball (Ni-Wan)

See Ni-Wan. Also translated as mud pill.

Mushroom of Immortality (Ling-Chih)
A kind of hard dark-brownish mushroom which keeps for a long time. It signifies long life and thus refers to the Embryonic Breath practice.

Nan Hua Ching 南華經
It is Chuang-Tzu. A major Taoist book attributed to Chuang Tzu (c.300 B.C.), who was called Nan-Hua-Chen-Jen in the T'ang dynasty (618-906 A.D.)

Ni-Wan 泥丸
The upper Tan-T'ien.

Non-action
See Wu_2-Wei_2.

One (The)
It refers apparently to the coagulated or gathered air in the lower Tan-T'ien.

Original Breath (Yüan-Ch'i)
It is also translated as primordial breath. See Embryonic Breath.

Pai-Hsing 百姓
A hundred surnames. The term generally refers to the people. In the texts here, it may refer to the joints and passes in the body.

Pai-Hu 白虎
See White Tiger

Pai-Ku 白姑
See Corpses.

Pao-P'u-Tzu 抱朴子
The style of Ko Hung. See Ko Hung. A book by Ko Hung. It contains two parts: Nei P'ien and Wai P'ien,

dealing with the practices of breathing, healing, prolonging life, politics and daily living.

Passes (The Three) (San-Kuan)
This expression refers to places where the internal energy is easily blocked. They are T'ien-Kuan (the heavenly pass) i.e. the mouth or sinciput (the upper portion of the cranium); Ti-Kuan (the earthly pass), the feet; Jen-Kuan (the human pass), the hands. According to the Pai Wen P'ien, the eyes, the nose and the mouth. See Homann, p.22, in Bibliography.

P'eng-Chiao 彭矯
See Corpses.

P'eng-Chih 彭質
See Corpses

P'eng Chu 彭倨
See Corpses.

Periods (The Four) (Ssu-Shih)
The four seasons. A five-day period was called a Hou. A three-hour period was called a Ch'i or Ch'i-Chieh (one of the 24 solar terms of the year). A six-Ch'i period was called a Shih (period or season). A four-shih period was called a Sui.

P'o 魄
The seven inferior souls which are the turbid spirits of the human body. They are called as: Shih-Kou (Corpse Dog), Fu-Shih (Latent Corpse), Ch'üeh-yin (Female Sparrow), T'un-Tzei (Swallowed Thief), Fei-Tu (Non-poison), Ch'ü Hui (Removing Dirtiness), and Ch'ou-Fei (Stinking Lungs).

Primordial Breath
See Embryonic Breath.

P'u 朴
>The Uncarved Block.

Receptacles (The Six) (Liu-Fu)
>They are: the stomach, the gall bladder, the large intestine, the small intestine, the bladder and San-Chiao (the three Cooking Vessels).

Ridge Vein
>The Tu vein 督脈 (or acupuncture channel) which begins at the lower end of the spine, goes up along the back to the rear of the skull, and ends in front of the upper lip, after having passed through the top of the skull.

San-Chiao 三焦
>See cooking vessels.

San Ch'ung 三蟲
>See Corpses.

San-Ku 三蠱
>See Corpses.

San-Kuan 三關
>See Passes.

San-Li 三里
>See Three Miles.

San-Ts'ai 三才
>The Three Powers, i.e. Heaven, Earth, and Man.

Scarlet Palace (Chiang-Kung)
>The middle Tan-T'ien, near the heart.

Sea of Breath (Ch'i-Hai)
>The lower Tan-T'ien.

Seven Injuries (Ch'i-Shang)
    See Ch'i-Shang.

She-Chi 社稷
    Gods of the soil and grains - one's country, the national altars.

Shih-Chieh 屍解
    See Deliverance from the Corpse.

Shih-Er-Ch'ung-Lou 十二重樓
    The trachea.

Six Receptacles (Liu-Fu)
    See Receptacles.

Ssu-Yin 司陰
    Director of the Secrets, residing on the left side of the mouth.

Ssu-Ming 司命
    The Arbiter of the destiny, recording man's wrong-doings.

Ssu-Sha 司殺
    The Executioner, residing on the right side of the mouth.

Sun and Moon (Re Yüeh)
    The left eye (also referred to as Shao-Yang) and the right eye (also referred to as T'ai-Yin).

Ta-Li 大曆
    766-779 A.D., one of the periods in the reign of Tang Tai Chung.

T'ai 胎
    See Embryo.

T'ai-Chi 太極
    See Grand Ultimate.

T'ai-Hsi 胎息
    See Embryonic Breath.

T'ai-Yi 太一
    It is the great Tao, the Absolute, the Ultimate One.

Tan 丹
    See Elixir.

Tan-T'ien 丹田
    Translated as the Elixir Field or the Cinnabar Field. There are three such fields: one above and in between the eyes; one at the level of the heart; one three inches under the navel. In these fields, according to Taoism, takes place the alchemical transformation of man into an immortal.

Tao 道
    The Way, The Path but also The Word. In the Taoist texts translated here, The One or TAO, it is equated with The Embryonic Breath.

Tao Te Ching 道德經
    A text of about 5000 Chinese words. The next most translated and interpreted (or perhaps it should be called mistranslated and misinterpreted) book after the Bible. Attributed to Lao Tzu. Usually interpreted as containing philosophical thoughts. Its secret interpretation in Taoism was with regard to breathing practices.

Tao Tsang 道藏
    A great anthology of Taoist canons, books and biographies.

Tao-Yin 導引
> Taoist gymnastic exercises designed to facilitate the retention of the breath and the flow of Ch'i in the body. A few of these exercises are described in detail in volume II of The Primordial Breath.

Te 德
> Translated as power, virtue or attribute. It may refer to the obtained realization of the Embryonic Breath.

Thatched Hut (Mao-Lu 茅廬)
> The nose, which is also called Shen-Lu (Divine Hut), Yü-Lu (Jade Hut), Ch'ang-Ku (Long Valley) or T'ien-Men (Heavenly Gate).

Three Miles (San-Li)
> The genitals. Sometimes it was called San-Hsing (Three Stars).

Three Powers
> See San-Ts'ai.

Three Superior Souls
> See Hun.

Ti-Hu 地戶 (Earthly Window)
> The mouth.

T'ien-Men 天門 (Heavenly Gate)
> The nose.

T'ien-Shih 天師 (Heavenly Teacher)
> See Chang Tao-Ling.

Tu Vein 督脈
> See Ridge Vein

Twelve Storied Tower (Shih-Er-Ch'ung-Lou)
> The trachea.

Vermilion Bird 朱鳥 (Chu-Niao)
　　The tongue. Also called **Gold Key 金鑰 (Chin-Yüeh)**

Vermilion Sparrow 朱雀 (Chu-Ch'üeh)
　　The heart. Also one of the four spirits residing in the four directions: the green dragon in the East, the vermilion sparrow in the South, the dark warrior in the North and the white tiger in the West. It has seven constellations.

Viscera (The Five) (Wu-Tsang)
　　See Five Viscera.

White Tiger (Pai-Hu)
　　A symbol for the lungs. See Vermilion Sparrow.

Window of the Earth (Ti-Hu)
　　The mouth.

Worms (The Three) (San-Ch'ung)
　　See Corpses.

Wu-Ching 五更
　　See Fifth Night-Watch.

Wu Hour 午時 (Wu-Shih)
　　11 a.m.-1 p.m.

Wu-Hsing 五行
　　See Five Elements.

Wu-Keng 五更
　　See Fifth Night-Watch.

Wu-Lao 五勞
　　See Five Diseases.

Wu-Sse 五色
See Five Colors.

Wu-Shih 午時
11 a.m.-1 p.m.

Wu-Tsang 五臟
See Five Viscera.

Wu$_2$-Wei$_2$ 無爲
The Taoist principle of Non-action. Though variously interpreted, the texts published here seem to use it as meaning the technique to stop one's breathing for a certain period.

Wu$_3$-Wei$_4$ 五味
See Flavors.

Wu-Ya 五芽
See Germs.

Wu-Yin 五音
See Five Notes.

Wu-Yüeh 五嶽
See Five Mountains.

Yang 陽
The male or positive element in nature, as contrasted with the Yin.

Yellow Court
The abdomen.

Yellow Court Canon (Huang-T'ing-Ching)
A Taoist work of high antiquity attributed to Lao Tzu. Its full name is T'ai-Shang Huang-T'ing Wai-Ching Ching. There is another book called Shang-Ch'ing

Huang-T'ing Nei-Ching Ching. Both books make the internal and external views of the Yellow Court Canon.

Yellow Peace (Huang-Ning)
See Huang-Ning.

Yi-Wen-Lüeh 藝文略
A general title catalog for Chinese classical books.

Yin 陰
The female or negative principle in nature; it is the opposite of Yang.

Yin Tan Pai Yu 陰丹百御
The Hundred Times Retained Yin Elixir. A Taoist secret practice of preventing ejaculation during intercourse.

Yü-Chen 玉枕
The Jade Pillow, the occiput.

Yü-Ch'ih 玉池 (Jade Pond)
The mouth.

Yü-Ch'üan 玉泉 (Jade Spring)
Saliva. Also jade dust to be mixed with dew gathered in a jade cup. The mixture allegedly was then ingested as part of the practice to attain immortality.

Yü-Lu 玉盧
Jade Hut, the nose

Yü-Shih 雨施
See Granting of the Rain.

Yü-Yeh 玉液 (Jade Juice)
See Saliva.

Yü-Ying 玉英 **(Jade Flower)**
   Saliva.

Yü-Ying 玉瑛 **(Jade Crystal)**
   Teeth.

Yün-Hsing 雲行
   See Cloud Practice.

Yüng-Ch'üan 湧泉
   The Gushing Spring. The center of the sole.

BIBLIOGRAPHY

BEIJING COLLEGE OF TRADITIONAL CHINESE MEDICINE, cmpl. Essential of Chinese Acupuncture, Foreign Language Press, Beijing, 1980.

CHANG Chün-Fang (張君房), ed., Yün Chi Ch'i Chien (雲笈七籤), Seven Bamboo Tablets of the Cloud Satchel. The Liberty Publishing Co.,Taipei, 1974.

CHAO Yung-Tsung
See Davis Tenney.

CHU Yün-Yang (朱雲陽), Wu Chen P'ien Ch'an You (悟眞篇闡幽), A Commentary on The Essay on the Understanding of Truth. The Liberty Publishing Co., Taipei, 1982.

DAVIS Tenney and CHAO Yung-Tsung, Chang Po-Tuan of Tien Tai, His Wu Chen Pien, Essay on the Understanding of Truth, Proceedings of American Academy of Arts and Science, vol. 73, no. 5, July 1939.

ERKES Eduard, trans., Ho-Shang-Kung's Commentary on Lao-Tse. Artibus Asiae Publishers, Ascona, 1950.

EVANS-WENTZ W. Y., Tibetan Yoga and Secret Doctrines, Oxford University Press, London, 1977.

GORAKHNATH Siddha Guru, Yoga Bija, Swami Keshwananda Yoga Institute, Delhi, 1978.

GUINESS BOOK OF WORLD RECORDS, Bantam Books, New York, 1987.

HOLMES Welch and SEIDEL Anna, Facets of Taoism, Yale University Press, New Haven and London, 1979.

HOMANN Rolf, Die wichtigsten Körpergottheiten im Huang-t'ing ching, Verlag Alfred Kummerle, Göppingen, 1971.

HOMANN Rolf, trans., Pai Wen P'ien or The Hundred Questions, E. J Brill, Leiden, 1976.

JAO Tsung-I (饒宗頤), Lao Tzu Hsiang Erh Chu Chiao Chien, A Study on Chang Tao-ling's Hsiang-er Commentary of Tao Te Ching (老子想爾注校牋) Tong Nam Printers and Publishers, Hong Kong, 1956.

KUO Mo-Jo (郭沫若), T'ien Ti Hsüan Huang(天地玄黃) Shanghai, 1947.

LI Hui-Li, Nan Fang Ts'ao Mu Chuang, A Fourth Century Flora of Southeast Asia. The Chinese University Press, Hong Kong, 1979.

MASPERO Henri, Taoism and Chinese Religion, The University of Massachussetts Press, Amherst, 1981.

NEEDHAM Joseph, Science and Civilization in China, University Press, Cambridge, England, 1954.

OFUCHI Ninji, The Formation of the Taoist Canon. See HOLMES Welch.

ROBINET Isabelle, Les Commentaires du Tao To King jusqu'au VIIe Siècle, Collège de France, Institut des Hautes Études Chinoises, Paris, 1977.

SASO Michael, The Teachings of Taoist Master Chuang. Yale University Press, New Haven, 1978.

SCHIPPER K. M., Concordance du Tao Tsang. École Française D'Extrême-Orient, Paris, 1975.

SEIDEL Anna, see HOLMES, Welch.

SHIH Vincent Y. C. (施友忠), The Taiping Ideology, Its Sources, Interpretations, and Influences, University of Washington Press, Seattle and London, 1972.

STUART G. A., Chinese Materia Medica, Vegetable Kingdom, Southern Materials Center, Inc., Taipei, 1979.

TAO TSANG (道藏), Yi-Wen Book Co., Taipei, 1962.

WARE James R., trans., Alchemy, Medicine and Religion in the China of A.D. 320 (The Nei P'ien of Ko Hung), Dover Publications, Inc., New York, 1966.

WIEGER L. Taoïsme, Librairie Orientale & Americaine, Paris, 1911.

WILHELM Hellmut, Eine Chou Inschrift über Atemtechnik, Monumenta Serica 13 (1948), pp. 385-388.

WU Sing Chow, A Study of the Taoist Internal Elixir - Its Theory and Development, University Microfilms International, Ann Arbor, Michigan, 1985.

YEN Ling-Feng (嚴靈峰), Wu Ch'iu Pei Chai Lao Tzu Chi Ch'eng (無求備齋老子集成), Yi-Wen Book Co., Taipei, 1965.

YIN Chen Jen (尹眞人), Hsing Ming Kuei Chih (性命圭旨),China, ca. 1700.

ZAPOL Warren M., Diving Adaptations of the Weddell Seal, Scientific American, New York, June 1987.